Life to be lived

Life to be lived
Challenges and choices for patients and carers in life-threatening illnesses

Catherine Proot
and
Michael Yorke

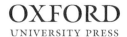

OXFORD
UNIVERSITY PRESS

OXFORD
UNIVERSITY PRESS

Great Clarendon Street, Oxford, OX2 6DP,
United Kingdom

Oxford University Press is a department of the University of Oxford.
It furthers the University's objective of excellence in research, scholarship,
and education by publishing worldwide. Oxford is a registered trade mark of
Oxford University Press in the UK and in certain other countries

Published in the United States of America by Oxford University Press
198 Madison Avenue, New York, NY 10016, United States of America

British Library Cataloguing in Publication Data
Data available

Library of Congress Control Number: 2013945061

ISBN 978–0–19–968501–1

Printed and bound by
CPI Group (UK) Ltd, Croydon, CRO 4YY

Foreword

There is optimism at the heart of palliative care

Cherny, 2007

This book is about life: life at the end of life. It is about helping people 'live their dying'. It is about the realities, messiness, uncertainties, the multiple contradictions, paradoxes, and ambivalence that are part and parcel of living through advanced illness, dying, and bereavement, but also about what helps and heals. It addresses the impact of advanced illness and intervention. It is based on volumes of experience of people who are distressed and in need of compassionate and skilled support. It is a masterful integration of the psychological, social, and spiritual, offering not only an understanding of these crucial facets of the holistic approach to working with people in end-of-life care, but also a response.

The authors focus on the 'life-altering' nature of advanced illness, end-of-life needs, death, and bereavement. Its richness is in the tone and approach of how you can treat people as full human beings, offering the potential and possibilities for change. It is the sheer humanity of the person affected and those supporting that speaks. The book is a strong reminder never to let slip that essential aspect of being with and working with ill people, needed in an increasingly medicalised world of healthcare, fast turnover of patients, and care rationing. Haraldsdottir (2011) in her research on 'being there' casts doubt on the practice of this mantra of many in the hospice movement. *Life to be Lived* tells how to 'be there' for people.

Life to be Lived is anchored in patient experience; it does not hold back on the realities of illness experience and the thoughts, feeling, and behaviours that comprise the experience of death and bereavement. It also addresses the experiences of those directly affected: family carers, local communities, health and social care professionals, and their organisations. It demystifies the complex, be it for the lay reader or experienced professional. We sometimes become anaesthetised to what is really happening in the wider world of the individual person and those who surround them.

The authors are to be congratulated on the method used to cover the material. The narrative research undertaken by Proot is used to best advantage by presenting the narratives and stories of patients, professionals, and others.

The abundance of these 'uncontaminated' accounts offer truths as well as signposts to professional and lay carers alike. From Veronica's diary extracts in the opening chapter: 'Is it possible that the cancer has recurred as a means of pushing me on and on down the road? If so what must I do to respond positively and *accept* the illness?' to Billy's detailed reflections of how he intervened as a social worker and family therapist to undertake quite complex work with a troubled family, or of a consultant, Jane's use of metaphor to help Naomi understand her cancer of the cervix. What speaks and teaches us is the weight of experience from the narratives in addition to the vast experience of the authors. They weave the theory through the practice.

This publication offers an inspiring way for people in contemporary society to re-view death as part of life. It complements the work of the Dying Matters Coalition and other initiatives for society and local communities to educate and free us from the fears and taboos surrounding death and to plan better. It is also a good response to government initiatives such as the End of Life Care Strategy (DH, 2008), with its emphasis on education and training the generalist workforce who come across the majority of people at the end of their lives. For them, this is a book on how to help people die well in their 'psycho-social-spiritual' space.

'People die alone in a very personal way, just as they live, and that the best we can do is to be there at the door if and when they can, or choose, to open it' (Chapter 15, 'In conclusion'). Thank you to the authors for telling us just how it is and how it can be. Above all, I welcome the fact that the pages in this volume speak of tenacity, the human spirit with its strength, resources, growth, and multiple examples of resilience in that 'psycho-social-spiritual' space.

David Oliviere
Director of Education and Training,
Education Centre, St Christopher's Hospice
September 2013

References

Cherny, N. 2007. Foreword. In: Monroe, B. and Oliviere, D. (eds.) *Resilience and Palliative Care. From Adversity to Achievement*. Oxford: Oxford University Press, p. v.

Department of Health 2008. *End of life care strategy: promoting high quality for adults at the end of life*. London: Stationary Office.

Haraldsdottir, E. 2011. The constraints of the ordinary: 'being with' in the context of end-of-life nursing care. *International Journal of Palliative Nursing, 17*, 245–250.

Preface

The writing of this book has been an adventure. In the course of its preparation, both of us have had significant spells in hospital, so we have examined our work with the critical eye of direct experience. The book, however, is not a personal testimony. We have learned much from others who have struggled with a range of illnesses, which in many different ways have been life-limiting for them. We have been touched by their courage and openness in sharing their experience with us.

This book is largely drawn from research and our clinical experience as a psychotherapist and a pastoral carer in bereavement counselling and palliative care. Our focus is people with a very serious medical condition that they know is almost certainly terminal or will probably be with them, if not for life, for a very long time. We refer to these conditions as life-limiting and life-threatening illness or, more generally, as life-altering illness, underpinning the profound impact that such illness has on people's quality of life and that of their relatives and friends. The stories recounted feature neurological diseases, heart conditions, diabetes, and strokes in addition to cancers. Most of the issues discussed are also relevant to other life-limiting conditions. The stress on carers, while varying at times in character, can be just as exhausting, difficult and isolating.

The book is written primarily for professionals and trained volunteers and those in training in the disciplines of palliative care. We feel its value lies in the highlighting of their non-technical role and presence. It may also be helpful to teachers and trainers in the field of hospice, palliative, and bereavement care and to patients and their families who wish to reflect on their responses to their situation.

The question considered is 'How do people face life-limiting illness and death?' This challenging and broad question, so significant to countless human beings, poses many other questions. We shall review a range of responses to illness and loss, the challenges posed to patients, relatives, and carers, and the support given, both personal and organisational. Most people need all the help they can get as they face these realities, especially when they are immediate and unavoidable.

We seek to be candid about the challenges involved for both patient and carer and to be frank about the limitations that are common in the care offered. We try to analyse what can bring a sense of 'healing' even when there is no cure.

What are the transforming processes that enable people facing life-altering illness to experience 'quality of life'? What helps or hinders the process? How can we foster improvement and the capacity to grow in adversity? We investigate these questions by exploring in depth and charting the experience of patients and families adjusting to and living with such illnesses.

The book highlights the importance of awareness and the significance of the attitudes and behaviours of those who are subject to major illness and those who care for them. The stories included are from actual accounts by therapists, chaplains, and patients. They are an important element in conveying our message, which we hope will be encouraging and inspirational.

We use personal stories to illustrate our points, but in order to protect the anonymity of our informers, all the names of patients and interviewees are pseudonyms and, where necessary to prevent breaking the confidentiality of third parties, settings are altered. Where gender is unclear we have chosen to refer alternatively to 'he' or 'she', or the use of the plural throughout the book in order to make the reading more fluent. The stories root our suggestions in living experience.

We have opted to produce chapters dealing with specific aspects and while they may be read on their own they contribute to a broad description of the experience. Our intention is not to prove anything but to contribute to a better understanding and appreciation of these times of transition for all the people involved, taking account of the specific contributions of social, psychological, and spiritual resources to this journey.

We trust that people involved in any way in palliative and end-of-life care may find in the challenges and narratives described in this book a repository of valuable resources to support and inspire their journeying with life-altering illness. Honouring the variety of ways to live one's dying and the fact that everyone's experience is unique, we hope that people may find here a set of messages that echo something of their own experience. They may be surprised to read it in the words of someone they do not know; someone who may even have died. Such discovery can be like a hand placed on one's shoulder. After all, we are not alone.

We hope that whoever reads this may feel valued and affirmed in their own experience and encouraged on their unique journey, in sickness and in health.

Catherine Proot and Michael Yorke

Acknowledgements

We are grateful indeed for the many who have contributed directly or indirectly towards the work. Among them we record our thanks to all the people who have made available their insights and experience; those who have checked the text; encouraged us to continue when the going became tough and gave us their advice and time. Among them we would like to mention by name:

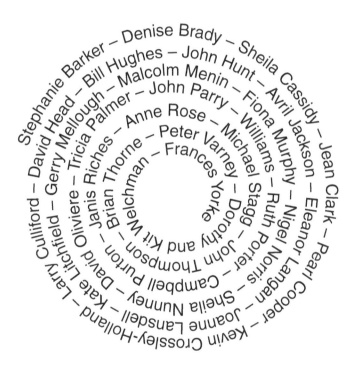

We would particularly like to thank Nicola Wilson and Caroline Smith from Oxford University Press and all those involved in the preparation and production of this book.

Introduction

The one certainty in our lifetime is that it will come to an end in death. We do not normally know when or how, and perhaps that is just as well. But for many, the when and the how does emerge because of serious illness or injury and such knowledge confronts us in many ways.

Death in many senses is the final taboo. In response, our society erects various barriers as a protection in order to remove the threat of death as far as possible, so that the joys and activities of life can be fully experienced and appreciated without such an ultimate distraction. One such device is the avoidance of talking about death, either by name or implication. When it is necessary, we frequently speak in hushed tones and use euphemisms such as 'passing away', 'falling asleep', or simply 'departing'. It would appear that some fear the very word because it brings the reality too close to their sense of being—or it becomes a reference to the unthinkable, the total ending of normality and their existence as people. Death is often perceived as a fearsome severance that must be psychologically repressed or denied. Such reticence in talking about death can create major difficulties, for instance in failing to make a will or discussing funeral arrangements. Our experience confirms that this failure to talk openly and make decisions about death and dying is common and leads to misunderstandings and disappointments at a time when sensitivities and emotions are particularly aroused.

Openness about death and dying is not deemed to be just a personal matter. Cultures themselves exert their own restrictions and requirements. Openness can productively and positively be assisted by cultural values and religious beliefs. If a culture has a sense of history, a pride in the past, and enthusiasm for the future, people can develop a realisation that they have a part to play in a long chain of endeavour stretching across the centuries and that they can contribute towards a better future. Religious beliefs reinforce the expectation that life is more than the immediate existence. The Abrahamic religions—Judaism, Christianity, and Islam—all teach about the reality of a future life in heaven or hell, even if these terms are not necessarily geographical identities. A confidence about the unknown future life seems consistent with the lessons of nature, of which humankind is a significant part, where death and rebirth form an almost universal pattern.

Such attitudes within a community have direct impact on individuals and families. Sometimes social contact is withdrawn, at other times there are flourishes of concern. Care and concern, apart from being intermittent, can be relatively short lived. People soon forget or downplay the bereavement of others, as they emphasise again their own concerns of daily living. Such experience can leave the bereaved lonely and vulnerable. They feel they are expected 'to pull up their socks' and 'get on with living' well before they feel ready for such a change of direction. We will consider the implications of these patterns of behaviour later in our book.

As we reflect on these issues, it is easy to perceive the confused thoughts and responses to the reality of death. Pervading the whole area is a strong sense of awe and mystery, which can provoke a fear of death and the power of its finality, together with a zeal for tradition that gives it dignity, while removing it from what we might term 'normal life'. It is probable that these contradictions reflect the widely divergent views as to what death really is and means. Is it the end of all things for an individual, or is it a doorway through which that individual moves to the next stage of life? Are the various religious teachings about death to be taken seriously as inspired revelation or are they the musings over millennia expressing unsubstantiated hopes? It could be argued that the traditions around dying and death suggest either a 'sitting on the fence' or a vivid recognition that all aspects of the process have a validity; thus thanks are offered for the passed life of the deceased, peace for the family and friends who mourn is requested, and hopes are expressed for a future life for the one who died. So we could conclude that many of the traditions and cultural expressions are efforts at containment of fear and provision of hope for another future.

The spiritual dimension, whatever one may mean by that, appears important in many cultures and we would affirm its significance for those caring for the chronically ill and dying and for the patients themselves, even where it does not extend to a belief in a personal life after death. How this comes into being and to fruition is one of the purposes of this book. John Swinton in *Spirituality and Mental Health Care—Rediscovering the Forgotten Dimension* (Swinton, 2001) reminds us that spirituality in its essence is indefinable. It therefore requires a willingness to accept uncertainty and mystery if we wish to work with it. However he points out that the effects of spirituality can be accessible and recognised in human actions and attitudes.

In spite of Swinton's warning about spirituality being indefinable, we feel that we must struggle to describe what we mean by the term because we use it so frequently in the text (e.g. in Chapter 12). Swinton describes the difficulty as mysterious, perhaps because it is 'differently common' to all human beings. It is an innate sense of another dimension to which we can aspire. Perhaps it is the deep driving force that helps people to understand who they are and what they can be. There is no common denominator, no norm—spirituality expresses itself, for good or evil, uniquely in every person. Thus strengths and weaknesses, hopes and fears, dreams or nightmares, ideals and plans, arts and science are signs that spirituality is at work in someone. As we acknowledge the descriptive difficulties in defining spirituality, its existence in the wider sense is identifiable. Putting into words these mysterious yet very important experiences in the field of palliative care is another of our purposes.

Religion and spirituality are often confused, but we are clear that, while frequently linked, they are not the same. Religion can be an expression of spirituality, but it is not automatically so. We like to work with the metaphor 'Spirituality is the hand; religion is the glove which fits it'. Each helps to define the other; fitting may be a difficulty and gloves can be changed or discarded, but hands are more expressive of the individual and the background which moulded them and thus would be the base of more enduring attitudes, priorities, and behaviour. A religious faith can be very important to many, especially at times of great uncertainty and vulnerability, and it can be the vehicle for personal support and care that would not otherwise be available. However a faith in God can itself be vulnerable and it is sometimes tested to breaking point in dire distress or threat, including major illness or impending death. Nevertheless, as we shall see, a spirituality, whether or not secured with a strong religious faith, can be a source of purpose, peace, and hope to those in such circumstances.

All the foregoing has indicated to some degree a public concern for marking a death appropriately, but also making sure that it is contained as a special but not over-emphatic part of life, even if it is inevitable. Such expressions as 'life must go on' and 'you will get over it in time' indicate at a deep level a desire to minimise the impact of major illness and death while still recognising its existence. For those immediately caught up by such life-threatening or life-limiting circumstances or even the death of a loved one, there is no putting aside their impact. For all concerned, patients and carers, friends and relatives, the experience is life-changing, temporarily or permanently. This book is an attempt both to indicate to professional carers and those in training the special challenges and feelings arising from their work with patients and families, and also to offer some ways for coping with them and learning from them. We will all one day die, but we hope our ideas will help us all, one day, to die well, whatever that may mean to us.

References

Swinton, J. 2001. *Spirituality and Mental Health Care—Rediscovering a 'Forgotten' Dimension*. London and New York: Jessica Kingsley Publishers.

Contents

Part 2 **The impact on family carers**

Part 3 **The professional carers and their roles**

Part 1

The patient experience

Chapter 1

The challenge of illness and pain

Everyone of us will have come into contact with a seriously ill person at some time or other. We may be sharply aware of the problem, even without any details, or not so at all, beyond having a vague sense that the person before us is not well. While we reflect on the fact of illness, it is necessary to remember that people react to illness in uniquely different ways, almost from the first realisation of a symptom to when advised of a diagnosis and beyond. As the recognition of the disease strengthens, so in some does a determination to fight it, if necessary to the death. Others will accept that they are very ill and begin to prepare for an uncomfortable period ahead and even for death. While physical symptoms and treatment will be uppermost in pursuit of a cure, illness also makes profound demands on and tests the emotional and psychological and indeed spiritual well-being of the patient and those they know.

Help me to live, not to stop dying

Our book relies primarily on talking to credible witnesses of the process of adjusting to chronic and life-threatening illness. We have been entrusted with a patient's diary—call her Veronica—with the kind permission of her widower and her therapist to use it for our purposes. We choose Veronica's direct voice, uncontaminated by any interviewer, to open this book and capture the flavour of what we intend to discuss. The narrative is extracted from her diary, which records her reflections during the first two of three years journeying with a recurring cancer. The emphasis is hers.

The most important health-enhancing thing is for life to be fulfilling, challenging, interesting, fun, worthwhile, changing, and growing. The more I understand about myself, the more I can achieve these things. Is it possible that the cancer has recurred as a means of pushing me on and on down the road? If so, what must I do to respond positively and accept the illness?

We cannot know about a God, but we can know we have a transcendent self. Do I experience my transcendent self? I can only explain it in terms of a love for people. It is some sense of connection with others.

What to think about faith and belief in relation to disease? Joanne (her therapist) told me of a Hungarian colleague whose reaction to Chernobyl was that when she went into the garden that day, the rain was tainted. Even nature was vulnerable—the thing she had always trusted. Like my body—I can no longer trust the valued, beautiful body.

Did I choose to be ill—unconsciously? God only knows, but I can choose to fight my illness while respecting it, not hating it.

Bone scan today. Feeling less well than I have recently, maybe the effect of the scan. Slightly nauseous. Felt so affected by seeing Joanne—had a sense of reviewing what is going on for me and we discussed how I have changed. Joanne follows my mood very closely, I think. She does not try to lift me, just stays alongside. The point is not to fix, to change or make it better, but to share the journey—an intimate journey; to create a safe environment to deal with the issues in life. Help people to live, not to stop dying.

Eighteen months later she writes:

Where am I on this journey? Who am I now? What do I need to do to travel further, explore deeper?

I feel I have let go of my fears of illness and death, but I cannot quite trust myself in this. What will happen if I really conclude that I have worked through the fear and pain and can let it go? It was there for so long, to teach me, to keep me working things out, being challenged.

I don't need it any longer. It has served its purpose well. What is the next stage about then? 'Growing in wisdom' can only be through experience and consciousness. Going deep into the experience—allowing whatever comes up to be there.

Pain

Many life-limiting illnesses include degrees of pain, and the physicality of cancer can overwhelm patients and carers. The problem of suffering and pain has haunted human beings and philosophical thinkers for thousands of years. All forms of pain are unpleasant, but most can be deadened by modern analgesics to the extent that they become bearable. However, there are still instances of relentless and/or continuous pain that people find exhausting and depressing. Pain can spring from a physical malfunction, but it can also indicate mental, emotional, and spiritual pressures, which can be hard to define and treat. It can be induced, for instance, by guilt, loss, anger, and many of the other strong emotions. It can be the expression of an undelivered or unheard message. Whatever its source, pain can be highly disruptive and destructive. Concentration can be lost, self-centredness and restlessness can grow. Pain often induces short-tempered outbursts and relationships can be very challenged. With ensuing anxiety and exhaustion, patients can feel 'trapped'; they are imprisoned and the key to release may be very difficult to find.

> Pain is not a simple affair of an impulse travelling at a fixed rate along a nerve. It is the result of the conflict between the stimulus and the whole individual.
> René Leriche
>
> Reproduced from Leriche R, *The Surgery of Pain* (Translated by A. Young), Bailliére, Tindall and Cox, London, UK, p.489, Copyright © 1939.

In spite of potential support through good and caring medicine and nursing, together with devoted family backing, for most people being ill is a distressing, frightening, and confusing situation. When things are not going well—as when the symptoms, fatigue, or drug reaction are mismanaged—the patient's anxieties are likely to increase along with an increasing dependence and helplessness. They are caught up in a great mystery far beyond them. They may feel an innocent victim, isolated without the understanding or empathy of others. Most of us, when fit and well, take our freedom to act with self-determination for granted. When we become ill, those freedoms seem to be taken from us: the doctor takes over, we have to become pliant, we are whisked into hospital, placed to sleep among strangers, nursed and handled by strangers who frequently appear to be overstretched and harassed. We feel lost and out of control. This is underlined perhaps by distressing symptoms of weakness, incontinence, and confusion. We lose the ear of those around us who are in authority and even the capacity and confidence to speak clearly. All we can do is to rage internally at our loss of identity and freedom, and feel shame at what we have become.

Such a scenario is tragic and distressing and works against recovery or healing. Very few instances of mismanagement or neglect are deliberate, but they do happen, if not at a physical level then often and all too frequently at a psychological one. They may well be caused by scarce resources, overwork or faulty attitudes, or by the carers' need to protect themselves emotionally. All tend to lead to the patient feeling that they are a case, not a person; a number on a medical record, and a statistic in a report. No wonder that, in such circumstances, we can lose heart and perhaps the health and the will we had. 'Healing' seems far away. But all is not lost.

Curing and healing

In the treatment of illness there are two dominant approaches to the process, often referred to under the general terms of 'curing' and 'healing'. The two traditions are frequently assumed to be the same, but we believe them, while complementary, to be different in method and goal. For most people, the aim is primarily to get rid of the symptoms causing the trouble with the goal that the patient will go back to who they were before the disease. The whole panoply of drugs, surgery, and nursing will be focused on that goal of survival. Healing, on the other hand, aims to create the right environment around the patient to encourage their own transformative and health-restoring processes. This will involve the emotional, psychological, and spiritual self, the immediate carers and the general environment in which the patient is placed. Healing is more widely focused on the whole person, with the goal of enhancing life, whatever that may mean. As Swinton (2001; p. 57) puts it:

> Healing is a deeply spiritual task that stretches beyond the boundaries of disease and cure into the realms of transcendence, purpose, hope, and meaning that form the very fabric of human experience and desire.

That suggestion coheres well with the notion that the process of healing leads the person to an experience of integrity and wholeness that springs from the inner core of the sufferer, which is that part that makes that person who he or she is (Dean's Working Committee on Healing, 2001–2003).

A sense of belonging, relationship, membership of the world, can grow as the healing balm is shared through the experience of love and warmth with those who care for them. Thus Michael Mayne, in his remarkable book *The Enduring Melody* (2006) in which he recalls his feelings as he underwent treatment for terminal cancer, notes how important were the relationships with his family and friends, with nature, music, reading and writing, and with the doctors and nurses who treated him sensitively or otherwise. He shows how he reacted when there was a threat to that sense of integration and relationship and how destructive it was for him.

Stress provoked by treatments

We referred earlier to the differences in people when they hear news of the nature of their illness, and there are similar huge differences in how individuals react to specific treatments, some mildly affected and others suffering considerably. Some see the treatment as a positive means to a cure, others will see it as an attack on their self-image and their personal significance. One could cite the example of the reaction to the loss of body hair following the use of some of the chemotherapies. While no one likes these side effects, some cope much better with them than others. As a wise country doctor used to say: 'There are no illnesses, there are only ill people!'

We live in an age of remarkable technical medical advances and deepening insights into human psychology and the struggles with stress, fear, and confusion. However, it is also true that many of the treatments available can have distressing side effects, which may cause acute unhappiness and physical and emotional disorder. Here lies one of the dilemmas for contemporary doctors as they make their decisions as to what to do when facing the important challenge of balancing the potential benefit of a treatment that can assist a cure with the negative effects that can go with it. Alongside the advances in treatments, there also lies the danger that scientific wonders and approach can be excessively influential and actually reduce the patient to an object to be cured rather than a person whose needs go well beyond the removal of a symptom. The determination is to make someone better, but what do we mean by that?

Psychological needs in treatment

Response to treatment not only depends on chemistry or biology, it is also conditioned by previous experience, by expectations and perceptions. It is even important that we like our physician, and certainly whether we respect and trust them. Similarly, if we had bad experiences with a doctor or dentist in the past, we are much more likely to be anxious or fearful, which in turn prepares us to react negatively in the present. Rabinovitch (2007) records in her diary that illness can 'lock us in' so that we become less able to look at an experience in a new way if negativity about it is already in place. Another example could be given: if we are put 'on hold', perhaps to improve assessment of our situation, some of us will accept that as a relief, others will see it as a dire threat. Some will perceive that things cannot be too bad, others will assume that there is nothing to be done; that there is no hope.

It is in these sorts of circumstances that the yearnings for loving care and encouragement are likely to be needed to help us to remain positive. While there is no general rule, those who do not have that support are much more prone to slip gradually into a deep sense of loneliness and depression. Others, being alone, will use it as an opportunity for constructive thought and focus on the invisible and spiritual powers that will help them to prepare for whatever may come their way.

Sometimes it is the very bad events that can be the lever to new spiritual growth. In a different set of circumstances, it can be the threat of divorce that leads a couple to really examine their marriage and make necessary corrections. Thus the deep need for tender loving care can trigger a new quality of relationship. On the other hand such emergencies can also indirectly cause the breakdown of relationships through stress and uncertainty.

These very personal realities remind us of a well known saying attributed to John F. Kennedy, who recalled that in Chinese the word 'crisis' is made up of two characters, the one representing 'danger', the other 'opportunity'. A patient-centred and holistic style of care could enable both these apparent opposites to be held and supported, giving the patient and their loved ones a sense of realism, but also of hope.

What is particularly threatening to the science of medicine is a sense of helplessness when there is no cure, and we need to ask what is 'healing' in those circumstances. Perhaps, in short, we need to emphasise the art of relationship in all its guises and to help people facing long-term and life-altering illness or death itself to experience the wholeness available in life, however that may be expressed for that individual. It is this important and life-giving process that produced the title of this book: 'Life to be lived'. We do not see the inability to cure all things as a defeat but as a challenge to advance medicine and care. Even when illness is terminal there is much rich, albeit at times difficult, living to be fulfilled, whether the dying process is long or short. When there is a sudden or catastrophic death, it is the loss of this precious time and space that is especially tragic. So we need to ask what are the supportive and threatening facets in this 'living space' in major illness.

Acknowledgements

Text extracts from Swinton, J., *Spirituality and Mental Health Care—Rediscovering a 'Forgotten Dimension'*, Jessica Kingsley Publishers, London and Philadelphia, Copyright © 2001, reproduced with permission from Jessica Kingsley Publishers.

References

Dean's Working Committee on Healing. 2001–2003. Montreal: McGill University

Leriche, R. 1939. *The Surgery of Pain* (Translated by A. Young). London: Baillière, Tindall & Cox, p. 489.

Mayne, M. 2006. *The Enduring Melody*. London: Darton, Longman & Todd.

Rabinovitch, D. 2007. *Take Off Your Party Dress. When Life's Too Busy for Breast Cancer*. London: Pocket Books.

Swinton, J. 2001. *Spirituality and Mental Health Care—Rediscovering a 'Forgotten' Dimension*. London and New York: Jessica Kingsley Publishers.

Chapter 2

All may not be lost

It has been unsurprising and comforting to realise that all is not entirely lost when a person's world is turned upside down by chronic or life-threatening illness. Relationships, values such as trust and hope, attitudes such as patience and humour, absorbing interests, and finding meaning further the process of coping with and adjusting to life-altering illness. An informant who has lived through cancer echoed Kissane's (2003) and Neimeyer's (2006) descriptions of the personal growth and positive reappraisal that can come out of adapting to loss:

> The illness was terrible, but I'm glad I went through it because I'm wiser; I know what's meaningful in my life and what is not. I take every day as it comes and think of it as a bonus. I'm more aware of other people going through similar experiences and I'm not so afraid for myself now. I feel more intensity of emotion, good and bad, but with a greater degree of equanimity, inner calm and peace.

This chapter looks more closely at what constitutes such experiences of positive reappraisal and growth.

Valuing patients as people

Illness can so easily lead us to think of ourselves as a case (and at times we are treated like one), but when we are treated as persons with feelings, hopes, fears, and opinions, these thoughts can be minimised, giving a sense of self-valuation: 'In spite of everything, I am still someone'. A feeling of integration contributes greatly to an awareness of safety, not just in a physical sense. It is not only the confidence in the drugs or the hospital, but an emotional safety arising from the experience of being held, loved, and cared for as a person.

It is the pursuit of such practices and attitudes that lead to 'healing' that lie at the heart of hospice care. Patients are people of value, of individuality, to be treated with respect, warmth, and touch. Even the most distressing and difficult treatments can be given in a manner that reduces stress and fear. The processes of feeding, bathing, and general care offered in an environment characterised by warmth, touch, and dialogue, provide an attachment quality similar to that of the mother–infant relationship described by Bowlby (1969, 1973, 1980) and Winnicott (1988). Similarly, talk, even about very serious and threatening matters, when put across with kindness, empathy, and the use of metaphor can be softer and more acceptable, without losing the core of the message. For instance, a discussion about the changing seasons and whether the bulbs will emerge can be used to talk of the process of dying, of change of circumstances, and of hope and trust in the natural cycles of nature.

Some personal sources of strength

Once again we remind ourselves of the crucial factor that always has to be remembered when caring for people: that we are all different and that facing major illness is an experience that will bring out these differences. Not only are our bodies and minds affected, but also our whole selves as a unity; our emotions, our perceptions, our hopes and fears, and our expectations and those of others for the future, including our dying. It is also important that we recognise that such differences of reaction will be found amongst carers as they seek to help those they love or those for whom they have responsibility.

There are many people suffering life-limiting illness who see things as a battle. They approach it in a spirit of determination, even in the face of a disease that generally brings early mortality or major disablement. They are determined to be the exception to the rule. Such patients can reveal remarkable qualities of courage, trust, and hope. Even when tested by pain and other trying symptoms, they continue to be strong outwardly and positive about the future. Such reactions can be fuelled by the determination to be present at a significant event, such as a christening, a wedding, a golden or a silver jubilee, or the birth of a baby, as in the following quote from Alice, a hospice chaplain:

> *Rebecca was quite poorly when she came in, but she was determined that she would be at her son's wedding within two weeks of her admission. Honestly none of us thought that she was going to make it, but she was determined to be in the photographs at her son's wedding. She made it. We didn't know how, she went to the wedding; she didn't even sit for most of the photographs.*

Defying logic, some patients fight very hard to remain involved in the world from which they are feeling excluded until something physical, spiritual, psychological, or social shifts and changes their perspective and health condition very quickly and unexpectedly. There is something that they want to see and they have decided to be there. And once they have done it, then they will die, but in their time, not in ours.

Another source of personal strength can be a sense of thanksgiving for life itself and all that has been received in the past. In the midst of prevailing pain, anxiety, and change of circumstances that major illness can induce, it is not easy to maintain a sense of thankfulness. It is hardly possible to be thankful for present trials, but if we can recall with thanks our past lives, positive gifts are made real. Thankfulness stimulates the will to look back over a whole life and how it developed and changed. It can be a humbling activity, but also a valuable and uplifting one, strengthening a sense of identity and achievement. Benedict, one of our informants said: '*The valuing of what was can give meaning to what is*'.

The recognition of order and process in our direct personal experience can help us, especially when facing long-term illness or death, to feel a sense of completion. This is fulfilling. It could even lead us, however surprisingly, to see our disease not purely as an enemy or a symptom to be overcome, but a lever to a wider understanding of who and what we are. This can bring a feeling of satisfaction and peace and, in turn, may facilitate an acceptance of what is happening, and its possible consequences. This can allow for unfinished business to be addressed, goodbyes to be shared, and where necessary reconciliations to be made.

Thankfulness can often be framed by a religious faith that gives a perspective to take the patient beyond the boundaries of life on earth. Such people may not be religiously active in terms of church membership, but they believe in an all-powerful God who guides and guards. This wider spiritual resource is evidently an important support for some in times of acute need. For whatever reason, many turn to prayer when things are perceived to be bad. When they feel powerfully threatened, they may find succour in holding a small cross or other significant symbol, not only as a release from their immediate fears but also, if they know others are praying for and thinking of them, as a reminder of their support and closeness.

Absorbing interests

In our experience of talking to carers and patients about their 'living space' in major illness, a number of supportive elements emerged frequently. In his book, Michael Mayne (2006) drew attention to the value to him of the discipline of writing. Veronica, whose diary is quoted at the beginning of Chapter 1, found writing it valuable because it assisted her power of self expression in trying to make sense of what she was experiencing. While reading and writing are not significant factors in many lives, they can give framework to existence when so many other facets of normal life are overwhelmed by pain and restlessness.

More generally, an absorbing interest can shift the focus away from suffering and helplessness. People may have very different interests of great concern to them, such as sport, gardening and flower arranging, or theatre and the performing arts, to name but a few. Absorbing interests can calm, uplift, and direct attention, while contributing to the all-important gift of a sense of involvement in the world.

Music and poetry, in all their forms, can be a much-valued resource. It is often said that music is a language that speaks to our emotions and souls and contributes to a refreshing equilibrium and restfulness amidst current chaos and confusion. People refer to the delight of watching nature—even in their garden, which becomes their wider world when they cannot get out. Alice, one of our informants, remembered a gentleman feeling bereaved because he had no garden to look at in hospital, so one of his grown-up children made him a card of a window looking through to a bluebell wood.

The 'music' of nature if it can be directly observed, even in a limited way, helps us to recognise the wonder of life and our share in it, in spite of our illness. The oft-quoted saying 'Say it with flowers' identifies the richness involved in floral beauty to the eye, touch, and smell. It is so sad that many hospitals now refuse their patients the gift of flowers for their bedside tables because of health and safety regulations and the extra work involved. It seems to us a denial of opportunity for the patient and of an important message of love, concern, thoughts, and hopes. On the contrary, many hospices enable patients to enjoy nature, even to the point of bringing in dogs and cats to see their owners and pushing beds out into the garden. They can enjoy the peace and normality as well as the beauty of these surroundings, to their great benefit and that of their visitors.

We see here how relief from constant reflection or concentration on the pain suffered or the inconvenience of disability can be valued by the patient, and also by the carers and household in general. Absorbing interests help all concerned to realise that not everything is lost. They can be instruments to lift the person from his present predicament so that they can be linked with other spiritual exercises, such as prayer or the love of nature.

Relationship and communication

We have mentioned the importance of valuing the person in relationships in the process of healing and also the restorative power of absorbing interests such as music, literature, and the visual arts. Communication of feeling and beauty lies at the heart of all these gifts, but it is the human contact, person to person, that is crucial, especially when one party is ill. This applies not only to the spoken word, but also to what is often called non-verbal communication, where information is conveyed by attitude and action. There is evidence (Bayliss, 2004, Fallowfield *et al.*, 2002) that the words we select to express our message deliver only a small part of our meaning. The bulk of it is conveyed by tone, volume, pitch, pace, and modulation of our voice as well as facial expression, body stance, and gestures. This explains why non-verbal communication, such as quality of touch and eye focus, is vital to our relationships at the bedside. Sometimes it can appear to contradict what is being said and thus creates confusion.

Non-verbal communication becomes even more important as patients' lives draw to a close. Towards the end, people are withdrawing; their field of awareness becomes smaller and the way in which they communicate becomes restricted. Being sensitive to their needs and what they are experiencing becomes increasingly difficult to read. Without interfering or throwing ourselves at somebody, it is important to use non-verbal ways of communicating as much as possible at this time, for instance through handholding and stroking.

Verbal communication involves information, facts, and data as well as feelings and perceptions. The doctor, nurse, or therapist may feel the need to compensate a little for lack of self-assurance in certain situations. The patient may laugh about some comments one day that may be quite challenging the next or when they are voiced in the presence of others. It is clear that when one is very ill, there is a real sense of vulnerability and dependence on others, so it is all the more vital that communication in all its forms is focused, kindly, and clear. It will not be the time for innuendo or cynicism, which can leave a patient confused and anxious, as in the following example taken from Michael Mayne:

> J. the radiation nurse, about to go on holiday for a fortnight in the sun [says]: 'see you two weeks on Monday—by which time you will be feeling really horrible!' Thank you, J. Among the things I neither want nor need to know, that rates pretty high. (Mayne, 2006 p. 215)

Those nearest to the ill person also may have problems of communicating with the patient or with each other. We consider this issue elsewhere in more depth, but the 'great unsaid', for instance that the patient is dying, becomes a sort of 'elephant in the room'. It inhibits both talking and behaving and allows urgent matters of what to do and who to deal with to be overlooked.

Supportive and/or challenging characteristics

Whether something is supportive or challenging can depend on the person. There are patients to whom staff struggle to give radio- or chemotherapy: their blood counts are never stable, their skin reaction is twice that of anybody else, they always have sickness and diarrhoea. Physically, they are not strong for one reason or another. Some people who are physically strong can be fragile emotionally, and this may lead them too to be unable to cope with the treatment. They do not have that inner strength that is required to persevere with a treatment that can be very tough. Their sense of who they are is threatened, their value to themselves and to other people is questioned, or it can be the fact that they do not care. When they feel completely valueless, they can see no sense in fighting.

People, both patients and carers, react to circumstances at any given time according to how they feel, physically or emotionally. If their mood is low and depressed, then they will reflect that in their reactions. Michael Mayne (2006), in commenting on the importance of contact with friends, recognised that he did not always welcome them because he might be feeling exhausted or frustrated.

Similarly, feelings and mood can affect the response to symptoms and pain. If the mood is low, the sensitivity to situations can be increased, with the sense of security or hope being undermined. Such variations therefore can affect the content and style of any support for all concerned. This demands awareness, flexibility, and tolerance—not easy requirements in such tough conditions!

The physical ordeals of increasing dependency, fatigue, and exhaustion are challenging, as are all ill-managed symptoms. As the illness progresses, loss of control comes in many forms: weakness, incontinence, confusion, loss of speech and movement, blindness, and the like. However, what is challenging or distressing does not necessarily have to be avoided; coming to terms with some difficulties is important and contributes to the process. We remember the story of the butterfly that was helped out of its cocoon by a compassionate little boy. The butterfly was never able to fly, because wrestling itself out of the cocoon was essential in strengthening its wings. What may seem the easier way is not always to the best advantage!

Acknowledgements

Text extracts from Mayne, M., *The Enduring Melody*, Darton, Longman and Todd, London, UK, Copyright © 2006, reproduced with permission from Darton, Longman and Todd publishers.

References

Bayliss, J. 2004. *Counselling Skills in Palliative Care*, Salisbury: Quay Books.

Bowlby, J. 1969. *Attachment and Loss, Vol. 1: Attachment.* New York: Basic Books and Hogarth Press.

Bowlby, J. 1973. *Attachment and Loss, Vol. 2: Separation, Anger and Anxiety.* London: Hogarth Press.

Bowlby, J. 1980. *Attachment and Loss, Vol. 3: Loss, Sadness and Depression*. Harmondsworth: Penguin.

Fallowfield, L., Jenkins, V. and Beveridge, H. 2002. Truth may hurt but deceit hurts more: communication in palliative care. Palliative Medicine, **16**, 297–303.

Kissane, D. 2003. Bereavement. In: Doyle, D., Hanks, G., Cherney, N. and Calman, K. (eds.) *Oxford Textbook of Palliative Medicine*, 3rd edn. Oxford: Oxford University Press.

Mayne, M. 2006. *The Enduring Melody*. London: Darton, Longman & Todd.

Neimeyer, R. A. 2006. Re-storying loss: fostering growth in the post-traumatic narrative. In: Cahoun, L. and Tedeschi, R. G. (eds.) *Handbook of Posttraumatic Growth: Research and Practice*. Mahwah, NJ: Lawrence Erlbaum, pp. 68–80.

Winnicott, D. W. 1988. *Babies and their Mothers*, London: Free Association Books.

Chapter 3

Trials and adjustment

Understanding the behaviour and thinking of the patient with a major illness is vital for the carer, whether professional or lay. In this book, the term 'lay carer' applies to those who are not professionally trained or do not work for any form of caring agency. It therefore generally covers family members, friends, and neighbours. The processes of adjustment can be difficult and threatening. This chapter describes some of the behaviours and feelings associated with these processes and how we can help patients and families in these difficult times.

Imposed change for most people is not welcome. It upsets our routines, our relationships, our economic security, and our expectations. The emergence of disease causes all these things and challenges patients' resources and resilience. It is therefore not surprising that illness, and especially serious illness, is seen as a major hindrance to a full life. However, some of the following stories demonstrate that this is not always so, even though illness is a tough testing ground for most of us.

Inner turmoil

When people are seriously ill, the questions 'Who am I?' and 'What am I?' frequently come to centre stage. Unless they can find some reasonably satisfactory answers to these questions life can be very challenging and difficult. Such questions as: 'What is my experience of this threat going to be like?' 'What will help me to deal with it and will I manage to do so?' 'Will I be up to it?' and 'What will I be like?' will underlie their responses to the changed situation.

Life-altering illness propels patients into a new and unknown world. Fear is overwhelming. They dread the illness and are full of uncertainty. Dina Rabinovitch (2007 p. 230) writes vividly of her anxiety, which makes her feel sick and breathless. She struggles to understand what these and other symptoms such as coughing mean. She wonders if she is relapsing. Even trivial things can be enlarged to become a problem and a threat, and patients may wonder 'Is this ache or cough "their cancer" or not? Is there hope for a cure? Should the doctor know about this? Is this a recurrence?'

Patients are anxious about their day-to-day experience of the illness and the treatment. They may over- or under-estimate a symptom. Whilst trying to cope with the new world of illness, they may also worry about their familiar routines. Perhaps they will ask themselves: 'Will I lose my job?' 'Who will look after the children?' 'How will I pay the bills?'

Immediate anguish about what one is feeling or what is ahead can be intertwined with deeper concerns for one's worth or value as well as one's identity. Alice, a hospital chaplain, tells of her encounter with Steven.

> *I went up to Steven on a ward round and said 'Excuse me, may I introduce myself?' He looked up, startled when he saw my dog collar, and started talking solidly for over half an hour. He didn't draw breath, I couldn't ask whether I could sit down, or get a chair. He just went on. I was wondering why I was listening to all of this twaddle, but another half of me listened between the lines to a very frightened man.*
>
> *A couple of hours later the ward sister bleeped me to go back and see him. He was due to go to another hospital for major heart surgery. He knew there was a very high risk that he'd not make it through the surgery and he was frightened, not unnaturally. He needed to talk. He had a lot to be ashamed of and feel guilty about in his past. He needed to do something about it and find a place of peace before he went off to put his life at risk.*
>
> *We sat in a quiet room for a couple of hours. He talked lots, and every now and again I reflected something back. He went off a very much more calm man and I wondered whether part of the reason he survived the surgery was that he was relaxed when he went.*

About to undergo major surgery, Steven was understandably very frightened. Despite a shaky start on their first meeting, he felt heard. This fuelled his trust and Alice, being with him and reflecting, offered him a space to talk. Feeling held, Steven could face his fears and confess his whole self—the nice and the not so nice things—in that one unifying encounter. He could be who he really was, and left a much more peaceful and relaxed man.

In contrast, fear and anxiety can produce anger: 'Why me?' 'What is happening to me?' 'It's unfair!' Alongside anger can come resentment and a sense of being picked on. However, when appropriately expressed, anger can be releasing, healthy, and positive. Even if it is releasing a frustration, many people still feel uneasy and confused about expressing anger. They may feel shame or embarrassment, numbness or depression.

Uncontrolled anger can be frightening, while partially repressed anger can be expressed in irritation at other people, impatience, grumbling, brooding, self-destructiveness, bitterness, coldness, and the like. Such behaviour can be a useful indicator of the patient's state of mind for carers, because it demonstrates the patient's inner turmoil.

Pain can be physical, mental, and spiritual. It can even be moral, when conscience is being disturbed or denied. There can be sadness about the illness and all that one becomes prey to. Some patients regret that they cannot fulfil their obligations and hopes, and this may lead to a sense of failure and loss of fulfilment in their lives. Working with patient Arthur in psychotherapy, Benedict was struck by how Arthur was journeying from a great deal of confusion, fear, and anger mingled with self-pity, towards a kind of reluctant acceptance, leading to a much more peaceful acceptance. It started with a sense of ambivalence about what he had been doing with his life.

> *What propelled Arthur to seek my help initially was that he was finding it extremely difficult to cope with his family and was experiencing significant ambivalence about the usefulness of what he had been doing with his life. He had invested much of his time, energy and life blood in his work, and, because of the particular work that he had chosen, in service of other people. Yet he was increasingly beginning to feel that his family members were comparative strangers to him, particularly his son.*
>
> *Questioning his life and relationships and adjusting to the illness were very much connected. No longer able to work, he lost his identity and his sense of direction and meaning deserted him. Becoming in many ways more reliant upon his family, from which he wanted relationship, nourishment and support, he began to realise that what he needed wasn't there; and the reason it wasn't there was basically his own fault.*
>
> *Arthur began to heal when he knew he was going to die. He had come to therapy feeling that his whole life may have been a terrible mistake and it was all too late to do anything about it. Once he knew he was dying, it was no longer too late. The death sentence somehow concentrated his mind and simplified the options. A new resolve and fresh meaning began to return to his existence, very different to what had previously been steering him. One thing only was worth doing: he must try to build a nurturing relationship with his family. He could let go of all the rest and almost give up on being regretful.*
>
> *Our relationship was also changed. What he was proclaiming he wanted to do was being paralleled in the therapy room. Up to that point Arthur had in a way fended me off. But once he knew that he was dying, he mellowed and became less distressed. He had an agenda which could now be implemented according to a new and different value system.*

Benedict has no doubt that the journey that Arthur made in those five months was incredibly important to him. A man who had arrived in total anguish and completely in pieces ended his life with a much greater sense of equilibrium and tranquillity, knowing that he had actually realised the goal he had set himself—to establish a meaningful and generous relationship with his family.

A cancer journey?

In reading and interviews, it is frequently noticeable how the notion of time has impacted on people's perceptions and experiences of life-altering illness in varied ways. The term 'journey' comes up repeatedly when speaking to patients and carers about healing, indicating a sense of duration and movement, forwards or backwards. Jane, a palliative care consultant and psychotherapist, speaks of the 'cancer journey', by which she means the lapse of time from the moment of suspicion that a person has a malignant disease through to the interview with the GP, then with the consultant, being told that it is cancer, and then treatment and the terminal phase. She remarked:

> Breast cancer treatment takes the best part of a year out of women's lives. Perhaps the process starts with them finding a lump, having a biopsy, leading to a lumpectomy and then perhaps another extended resection; about a month later chemo may start which could go on for six months; and a month or later maybe radiotherapy begins and may last for six weeks.

Taking a year out of people's lives brings disruption and alienation, not to mention how people change during that period. They often feel that they cannot go back to the life they left a year before.

The 'journey' metaphor suggests a point of departure and a destination, and maybe some stops along the road. These are not clearly defined, yet people's 'felt sense' of movement is expressed in the metaphor. Such a sense of movement may underpin the use of the term 'journey to acceptance'. Benedict, a counsellor, reflects:

> The process of healing as I would conceptualise it, is something to do with a journey. It represents a movement from confusion and feelings of hopelessness and helplessness to a sense of acceptance. At first, it is often a form of resignation and reluctant acceptance, which can, with time, grow into a greater sense

The 'felt sense' is a technical expression from the focusing method (Gendlin, 1981, 1996, 1997). Rooted in a profound philosophical analysis of the relationship between experiencing and symbolisation (Purton, 2004 p. 185), focusing helps people grasp the whole of an experience, sensation, colour, feeling, etc.

of inner peace. What is standing out for me is the struggle to make sense of it all.

Jane, too, recognises a patient's journey to acceptance. She said that she felt patients are moving towards acceptance when they become more peaceful and less desperate for a cure. In women with breast cancer a lot of shame and sexual connotations are tied up in their body, their identity, and how they look. Such feelings take time to be assimilated. It is indeed a journey, in which people move back and forth between signs of grief—shock, denial, anxiety, and panic—and periods of acceptance or recovery. Jane had also noticed a moving on to some form of withdrawal:

For a young woman to die and leave her children is unbearably hard. When some women have accepted that death is imminent they don't want to see their children towards the end because it is too painful for them. So a few days before they die, they withdraw from their children. I found this very hard to understand initially, but then I could see that it was the only way they could cope without going wild with grief.

Hearing about the withdrawal of young mothers from their children is heartbreaking, and yet so understandable from the perspective of a woman trying to protect herself from unbearable grief. In these moments it seems essential, if possible, that carers and members of the palliative care team offer husband and children an explanation for what is going on, so that the rejection by the mother may be made more bearable.

Longing for normality and yearning for safety

Several times in this book we mention the fear and anxiety so generally aroused in patients at the onset and in the course of major illness. These feelings arise from physical factors associated with being ill, such as the impact of anaesthetics, pain or discomfort, investigations, and disruption of what was for the patient and his family normal life. There is also psychological pain caused by not knowing what is to happen, the separation from loved ones when in hospital, and experiencing powerful and new dependency on unknown doctors and medical staff. Patients can feel that their life is being taken over and that they are powerless.

For some, such feelings are in themselves an ordeal. They lose the capacity to express themselves, cannot sleep and go off their food. They yearn for normality to return and they yearn for safety as they look forward to a very uncertain or changed future. As a patient once said to one of us: 'Please get me out of this place!' He was talking of the hospital but he was using 'this place' as a metaphor for his illness. He was really pleading: 'Please get rid of this disease'. Sadly the visitor could not respond with a miracle or a piece of magic, but the yearnings for change were powerful.

The longing for normality as previously experienced could be thought of as normal. Patients yearn for a return to their usual family life, routine, and work patterns. In those, they felt there was security, and a degree of certainty and stability. The illness is felt to have attacked these fundamental assets as well as the body or mind. The yearning can be, to a degree, illusory. The past can be imagined to have been secure, certain, and stable, but in reality it may not have been, and never is in total. We live with unknowns, tragedy, accidents, and negative changes, but yearning can overlook this fact. For the patient, while seemingly finding comfort and perhaps a source of thanksgiving, the past in all its facets can be enhanced to a perfection that is hardly possible. At the same time, the presumption of perfection emphasises the grimness of the present, and this can understandably have a negative effect on the patient's morale. The capacity to cope can be undermined, and attention to what is and needs to be done can be distracted, which does not assist in the circumstances.

Yearnings do not only apply to the past; they can significantly affect the responses to the future. The yearning for safety and security in the face of a perceived future threat can lead to a denial of what will or could be and an escape from a degree of positive cooperation. This could be vital to the patient's restoration to better health and well-being. Cooperation by the patient is important to medical practice and their attitude contributes to this positive approach. It is natural that patients are concerned for their future and long for the assurance of the good care, encouragement, and appropriate skills that can lead to a sense of safety, but the longing should be realistic and supportable and not based on delusion or fantasy.

Family and friends can assist considerably in helping the patient to a proper balance in their deeply held desires and needs, just as they can help in more practical ways by regular visiting and loving care. Similarly, the professional's recognition of the importance of yearnings will contribute to their deeper understanding of where the patient is.

The Liverpool Care Pathway for the Dying is a holistic care plan applied in hospices, hospitals, and increasingly in Primary Care Trusts (PCTs) as soon as the dying process has set in. Aiming to provide maximum comfort and support, it consists of hourly multidisciplinary checking and adjusting of the physical, psychological, spiritual, and social well-being of the dying person and their family. In the process of implementing the Liverpool Care Pathway for the Dying in a PCT, nurses and non-medical people were asked what they considered to be 'a good death'. The nurses' first answer involved symptom and pain control. Contrasting to this, and strikingly, the families and patients prioritised safety, privacy, and dignity. This confirms our conviction that these aspects should lie at the heart of what we, as carers, offer to those we serve.

Jane used to involve a teddy bear, Gus, to help to further a sense of safety in her patients.

> *Cathy's breast cancer had recurred and she was very frightened. She had a rather distant relationship with her husband and she used to come to me once a week for counselling. One week she was obviously suicidal. I was worried and rather than calling the psychiatric people in, which I knew she would hate, I persuaded the ward sister on the oncology ward to admit her. I went home leaving what I thought was a job well done, only to be rung up at 10 o'clock telling me that Cathy was discharging herself.*
>
> *I drove to the hospital clutching Gus, my bear, and sat and talked to her. After a while I said 'I will leave Gus to look after you'. She grabbed hold of him, shot under the bed clothes, and pulled them all over her head. In the morning I came to the ward and there was this hump on the bed. Eventually she emerged, clutching Gus. I said 'I think Gus had better go home with you'. He did and came back, by post, the following weekend in a brown paper parcel.*

The comfort Cathy found with Gus is similar to that of a child who cannot part from a piece of blanket or a cuddly toy that represents home and mother, and therefore safety. Gus worked as a transitional object (Winnicott, 1953), i.e. an object that linked Cathy with her therapist and made her feel safe.

Attachment theory (Bowlby, 1969, 1979, 1980) teaches how safety and security can grow and develop when the mother is recognised as a secure base from which the child can journey out to explore the world, knowing that it can come back to a safe haven in times of threat. People with a life-altering illness are extremely frightened, and the hospice, the therapist, or the care team can become such a secure base. They know that they will receive adequate care, that they will be understood, and that someone will not shy away from what they are experiencing. They feel held. Staying close to patient's experience in this way requires courage on the part of the people who work in this caring environment. Herein lies a great challenge for our major hospitals.

The yearning for safety not only focuses on external factors and what is received from outside oneself, but also one's own inner sense of self-confidence. This involves personal boundaries and where they are drawn. Privacy and dignity are challenged by the increasing dependency that often accompanies life-altering illness. At times, the statutory demands to secure privacy require too much of the patient, for example having to shower or bath themselves or even using the toilet when they do not feel up to it. Some people readily accept being taken care of. Others are inclined to rise to the challenge of doing all they can themselves, even if it costs them precious time or fatigue. One patient made it a point of honour, each time when in hospital, to dress in the morning, wrestling with the connected tubes and drips. Benedict's patient Arthur had a similar inclination:

> *Arthur was a big man and it was obviously painful for him to climb the stairs. When I suggested going into one of the downstairs rooms he said 'As long as I can clamber up these stairs, I am coming up here'. He wasn't going to unnecessarily capitulate and let go of his dignity and power.*

Even though Benedict was trying to be helpful when he suggested meeting in a downstairs room, Arthur would have none of it. He intended to hang on to the little control he had as long as he could. It was a matter of dignity, and perhaps also of fear that he might never retrieve any capacity he gave up. Safeguarding privacy, maintaining such discipline, can give a sense of control and self-worth. On the other hand, dignity and self-determination can include being willing to hand oneself over and to accept help. Thus the time came for Arthur when illness did take over and he had to tap into other resources.

> *In his last fortnight there was no dignity left and Arthur had to contend with that. What helped him to do so was that his family was able to come in to see him and be with him. He had pulled it off somehow. His family honoured him for it.*

To see the physically and socially powerful man that Arthur had been five months before, weak and dependent in a hospital ward, was challenging for Benedict, his therapist, who empathised with Arthur's sense of humiliation and loss.

Arthur shows that where emotional, spiritual, and physical needs are met, the pressures upon a patient's sense of being himself can be alleviated. His yearnings for recognition and integrity are met and he can find a new peace that is real and which conforms to his yearnings for safety and security.

A network of support

Patients do not live in a vacuum, and how they manage to cope with and work through the ordeal of chronic and life-threatening illness is influenced by many experiences around them: in the family, in the hospital, and in wider social networks. When people start treatment they enter a new world, with its challenges and routines and the support and companionship that they experience during this time.

When they are in the hospital, patients are in a total state of dependency. When they go out, there is a sudden loss of the dependency they have come to rely upon so much; hence the anxiety. There is more than the illness. The dependency is transferred and they have lost a bit of themselves too. It is about their state of being, their state of life. The framework is gone and patients are pushed back on themselves. This anxiety is theirs, but also that of their partner and family. The individual cannot be separated from the framework. When there has been a massive change, which can alter the structure in which relationships are experienced, family bonds may break down as a consequence. A therapist reflects:

> *Recurrently there were issues in their own journey: 'I've had a wake-up call, what do I want to do with the rest of my life?' or in the relationship with their partner or family. There was often little space for partners to say: 'I don't know how to help and I don't know whether it is okay to say I'm frightened too! You might die, and I don't really know how that feels. I don't know how to say this, I don't want to upset. I have to be the strong one and do the looking after and actually, I'm not keen.'*

Within the unknowns brought about by illness, projections and assumptions creep in between patient and partner. Counselling can help to clarify these and clear them out. The patient, for instance, can say and be heard in 'I felt you wouldn't listen when I said I was scared I'm going to die' and the partner in his response 'I couldn't bear to hear that, I was really scared you were going to die too'. Counselling may help to establish more open communication about fears and feelings and thus reduce anxiety and helplessness. It can also improve the partners' sense of mutual dependency in changing circumstances.

During treatment the hospital environment takes centre stage in patients' lives. A great amount of time is spent with nurses, doctors, therapists, volunteers, ward neighbours, and their families. They are often the first resort for questions to be answered and anxieties to be shared, as well as for mutual support and understanding. It is a striking transition from being well to becoming ill and having to fit hospital appointments into one's life, which is turned upside down by it. Autobiographies of cancer journeys are full of examples of how control is taken out of patients' hands. Rabinovitch (2007 p. 171) felt she was regressing from being an independent adult in control of her life to what felt like being a dependent child relying on other peoples' knowledge and expertise.

As one starts getting used to the cocoon of the hospital environment, it is suddenly over. The patient can miss all the companionship he found in the hospital, he may yearn to be close to his doctors. Any excuse to ring them can be grasped, for the familiar voice provides a sense of being closer and safer. Sue, who worked as a radiographer and a therapist, had a striking story:

> While people were being treated they were fine, they saw a consultant every week and they had the same nursing staff. They felt cosseted and cared for. At the end of their treatment we said, 'Okay, Mr Smith, come back and see us in a month! If you have any problems, give us a ring, but your next appointment to see us is a month after your treatment finishes.'
>
> Boyd, a bank manager, and his wife both said to me that that first month was a nightmare. He was looking at himself and wondering whether he was all right. She was looking at him wondering, what do we do? How do we manage this? What happens now? They had three months, or six months of their lives completely turned upside down, completely controlled by a process that says 'You turn up here', 'You have this treatment now', 'You have three weeks' gap'. And there are all these people to talk to, to reassure you, and at the end somebody pulls the rug out and says, 'Off you go!'
>
> Boyd and his spouse found that very difficult. They also found it very difficult when they had a cold, or other normal things, to be able to judge whether this was okay. Did Boyd take paracetamol? Did he go to bed for two days? Was this recurrence?

For months, patients are being told what to do at every step of the line. This can feel disruptive but also very supportive. They are closely monitored and meet the same nurse at every appointment, to whom they can talk about all the little worries that may or may not be linked to the treatment, and he or she can reassure them. They feel held by the staff companionship; a holding which, as we have seen, has attachment qualities to it.

On discharge from hospital that safety, support, and reassurance is suddenly taken away. Patients are back into 'normal' life, on their own, with the additional anxiety of whether they dare to trust their body again. The patient faces a further new situation: in spite of going back to the familiar setting many questions linger in the mind: 'How will I cope?', 'What will be my reception at home?', 'Will they understand that I feel different?', 'How will they care for me?' 'Will they pity me? Boss me about? Be curious and intrusive?' Fears do not decline on discharge; rather they can increase, eventually to the point of threatening patients' home relationships. They stem from the patient's physical and psychological weakness. To some degree patients are thrilled that they are going to be discharged, but underneath there is anxiety about whether they will be able to cope. They may be worried about becoming the subject of gossip, or having too many visitors who stay too long and wear them out.

The professionals need to be aware of these issues and remember that even small words of encouragement can make a big difference.

References

Bowlby, J. 1969. *Attachment and Loss, Vol. 1: Attachment.* New York: Basic Books and Hogarth Press.

Bowlby, J. 1979. *The Making and Breaking of Affectional bonds.* London: Tavistock.

Bowlby, J. 1980. *Attachment and Loss, Vol. 3: Loss, Sadness and Depression.* Harmondsworth: Penguin.

Gendlin, E. T. 1981. *Focusing,* New York: Bantam New Age.

Gendlin, E. T. 1996. *Focusing-Oriented Psychotherapy. A Manual for the Experiential Method.* New York and London: The Guilford Press.

Gendlin, E. T. 1997. *Experiencing and the Creation of Meaning. A Philosophical and Psychological Approach to the Subjective.* Evanston: Northwestern University Press.

Purton, C. 2004. *Person-centred Therapy. The Focusing-oriented Approach.* Basingstoke: Palgrave Macmillan.

Rabinovitch, D. 2007. *Take Off Your Party Dress. When Life's Too Busy for Breast Cancer.* London: Pocket Books.

Winnicott, D. W. 1953. Transitional objects and transitional phenomena—a study of the first not-me possession. International Journal of Psychoanalysis, **34**, 89–97.

Chapter 4

Towards a changed outlook

Many people when confronted by illness are shaken by its sudden onset or the gradual deterioration from what they considered their normal selves. The struggle to make sense of it all can be an important constituent of healing. It can promote discussion and a review of the relationships and the values that had been essential in the past. This process can lead to a sense of hope and a patience to wait and see. Such discussions also could become a means to that most precious of gifts when things are bleak: a sense of humour and lightness of touch.

When their life has been shaken up, patients with chronic, progressive, and life-threatening illness may discover new patterns and new meaning to life, which seem to sustain them. Many say that they see the world in a different way and their priorities change. Victor Frankl (2004), with a typical poetic note, points to how the way a person accepts the ups and downs of their life and their consequences gives them the possibility, even in very difficult circumstances, to find a new and deeper meaning to their life. Some patients almost feel grateful for the illness, appreciative of what they have discovered through it. Even if the result is negative, as in 'This happened to me because I have had an affair' or 'because I am a bad person' or 'because I did not go to church', finding meaning for themselves in that gives them a hold on what is happening. The value of discovering some meaning in the midst of illness is more important than the negative aspects of what they discovered. Family therapist Billy reflected:

> *Somebody who was attacked and suffered post-traumatic stress disorder said to me three months later 'I've discovered it was a brilliant opportunity because I have decided to move house, which I spent ten years thinking about'. Others say 'I know who my friends are now' or 'My family has been marvelous'. One woman said to me 'I am ready to sail out of my harbour'. I think I know what she meant. She wouldn't have chosen to die, but she had prepared herself for the journey.*

These are sentences that people have said, indicating that they had shifted their world view from chaos and crisis, from 'I don't know how I can cope', to 'Every day is a bonus'. The stories in this chapter bear further witness to patients' changes in their perception of themselves and others as a result of what has happened to them, and to how creative and determined they can be in trying to make sense of it all.

The part of life one has not lived

It has been said that when the end draws near, people are less regretful about dying than about what they have missed out, including the things they have not lived and experienced. Carl Jung (1992) speaks of how, in the process of 'individuation', people in the second half of their lives enhance their less-developed attributes. The following stories are examples of how ill people may experience healing when they have the opportunity to develop that other side of themselves and to be able to give voice to the part they have not lived.

Hopes and ambitions, so important before the illness, become less pressing and can be replaced by efforts to enrich what has been but is still incomplete. A realism may set in about what might have been undertaken, but also a realisation that no-one can do everything: 'My identity is based on what I am and have done, not on what I might have been and haven't'. But new good things can still be achieved, in spite of or perhaps because of the present situation, tough as it is.

> Doris, a patient, gives us an example of courage and unselfishness as she offered befriending to other people who were also suffering. Profoundly crippled for the whole of her life, she spent her final years as a practising Christian, praying for other people in need, and welcoming other residents in her home to talk to her in her room. At her funeral, she was described as a latter-day saint.

Addressing the part that has not been lived can give a sense of completion, which in turn gives meaning and purpose to people who are dying and supports their families after their death. More particularly, a sense of fulfilment in wholesome and mutual relationships supports or gratifies the dying person and can help the grieving process of those who are left. Charles, a Jungian

I wept for the lost opportunities.
I wept for the lost moments of happiness.
And in the end I wept for the lost companionship.

Philip Gould

Reproduced with permission from Gould, P., *When I Die: Lessons from the Death Zone*, Atom, an imprint of Little, Brown Book Group, London, UK, Copyright © 2012.

therapist, speaks of the spiritual quality of Ella's journey, recognising and developing parts that allowed her to come to life.

> *Ella was the wife of a distinguished army officer and a man who spoke little. When he retired, he withdrew into himself. Ella had hitherto filled her life with travel and making and meeting many friends. These relationships stimulated her.*
>
> *As she grew older, arthritis began to restrict her movements, and she gradually became isolated and lonely. Her comfort was to hold in her hand a small silver box, which she had acquired when she was at boarding school. When her husband died, her arthritis eased a little and she was able once again to get about. In the winters she travelled to warm climates and renewed friendships with artists and musicians. Life for her was being restored. One of her friends gave her some polished stones, which like her silver box gave her comfort and assurance.*
>
> *At a low time, she met Charles, a counsellor. She regaled him with her stories and through them began to live again. As a result of her memories, Ella lost some of her fear of death. She developed a new meaning to her life and accepted that she was not going to be a hero like her husband or famous like some of her friends. She found and accepted her place in life, however modest that may be.*
>
> *A few years later Charles received a call from a relative of Ella, saying she was very ill in hospital. She had heard Ella using Charles' name and they assumed she wanted to see him. Ella had been in a coma and hadn't spoken, eaten, or drunk. Charles went. He remembers 'She was just lying there, in a room on her own. While I was sitting at her bedside, I was quietly meditating a bit on God, or love and kindness. Suddenly, she sat up, bolt upright, opened her eyes, looked at me and said 'You've come. I just wanted to say thank you'. We both cried, she lay down, I left and she died'.*

This story is so powerful that it seems almost inappropriate to comment on it. Towards the end of her life, when arthritis was limiting her scope of action, this lady had found a way to come to life. The recognition that she was dying could be tolerated more easily. Ella's story is a striking example of how a life's journey tends towards completion and fulfilment despite and through limiting circumstances. Ella had experienced much of her life almost as an unlived life. She did not know how to connect with her spark, and was uncertain about how to express herself. But she did not stop trying and, in the last few years, could experience coming alive. There was a connection after all. Charles reflected:

> *Ella was a person waiting to be born, and yet could not get born. Her spirit could not somehow do what it had to do until relatively late in her life when it*

could also communicate with me and through her in a way that was significant and necessary. So it was in the end giving me far more than I had ever given her. It was a revelation in my experience.

With Ella it seems that her experience of her illness and her work with Charles led to the recovery of her ability to live. This experience suggests that in order to know how to die well we need to know how to live well. She could not die without having lived, but having learned from and responded to the constraints and life changes of her illness, she was in some way prepared for death when it came. As her therapist suggests, there was a spiritual quality to Ella's transformation. That she seems to have come out of her coma to thank her therapist is incredibly moving. Her story bears witness to the mystery of what we are dealing with. As a privileged companion, the therapist or carer can watch and be present, but they are not responsible for a transformation that goes far beyond what they can offer, even if what they offer contributes to creating the space for such a transformation to occur.

Discovering meaning

Some patients discover the meaning of their life by carrying out a full review of what they have been and done and what their journey on this earth has been like. They take stock of what has been significant, revisit places they have liked, and clear unfinished business. Eve, a hospital chaplain, tries to help people to recognise the purpose in their life. Asking about what they have lived and experienced, the good and the not so good memories, she finds that patients often talk about the things that have shaped them. Robert's story highlights the importance of relationships in this, particularly within the family:

Robert knew he was facing death and I was asked to go and see him by the palliative care team. He was longing to talk, even though he didn't want to talk about religious things. He had two sons who didn't live close to each other. However, through Robert's illness, they found that they could make time for each other. They started meeting up and motorcycling together. This was very satisfying to Robert, and he longed to tell me about the experience. He realised that it was very important to him that they got along. Deep down, it may have been the prospect, quite unarticulated, that he'd soon leave this family that enhanced his sense of significance that the two boys were close. It helped him face more easily leaving the world.

Seeing his sons get along helped Robert to leave this world with some contentment. Their newfound support for each other, something he felt important for their future, was ensured.

Many informants reported that where a relationship had been (or became) good and mutual, the letting go became easier for the patient. Surrendering and parting are still very painful and there is likely to be grief and distress, but when relationships are open and healthy, it becomes more of a natural process. The opposite may also be true: that if grief and distress do not pass, it may be an indication that relationships were not so good and/or there is some unfinished business.

Counselling, while allowing people the space to reflect on their lives in general, can also help them to perceive a meaning in their situation. The crisis that illness brings into peoples' lives may open up space for reflection and change and this is sometimes experienced as very intense and fruitful, despite the ordeal. Empowered to reflect and make their own choices, some people facing the uncertainty of life-threatening illness suddenly manage to sort out a number of things and come more to grips with their own lives. But sadly this is not always the case. Ria stands out in Jennifer's memory as a disappointment and an example that not all counselling is a success:

In her late forties, Ria had had a series of unhappy relationships, but she'd met someone on the Internet who she got on very well with. He had family, was divorced and had custody over the children. When Ria started going out with him she had to spend a lot of time in his house with the children present. One of the children was very hostile to her and she felt she wasn't getting enough attention. She missed spending time at home with her pet cats.

Ria couldn't decide: did she want to stay with that man who was nice and very attentive when they were together, or should she leave? But could she leave? She felt she was damaged; she had this cancer that might come back and would she find anybody else? Having this struggle, Ria wanted me to tell her what to do. She kept asking me to be honest, saying she didn't know what to do.

Ria was afraid of being alone, and we talked about some of the things that she could do. She had friends that she could go and visit, start doing things on her own. We tried various ways to look at her issue and then she stopped coming because, I think, I wouldn't give her what she wanted, which was to tell her what to do. It was disappointing that she stopped coming.

Some patients/clients want to be told what to do. This runs contrary to the principles of good counselling which seeks to support the person in taking responsibility for themselves and their decisions. Despite Jennifer's efforts, Ria chose not to come any more. This was disappointing for the counsellor.

As a therapist Chloe believes that narratives are important in building resilience. Her interventions are adapted to the story being given to her. If patients go into 'things are terrible and life is terrible' mode she may look for that one time when it was not so awful and try to build that up rather than focusing on the dominant story about life being terrible. Jennifer, a person-centred therapist, allows patients to listen to themselves, to discover the meaning of their ordeal and how they deal with it. She feels it is rewarding when patients or clients realise their difficulties and they are responding normally. By allowing them to talk about things, she finds that people recognise some ways to address the difficulties and challenges or learn to accept and live with them.

As we have noted earlier, some patients engage in a form of life review. They want to tell their story and talk about the things that they are proud of and what they have done really well, but they also want to talk about some of the things about which they may feel some degree of regret, guilt, or shame. It is almost as if they are trying to evaluate the balance of their life, which seems a really important thing for some people to do. This can be challenging for the listener, who may be tempted to minimise the negative and amplify the positive to try and make it sound better. Most of the time, however, when reviewing their life people are almost talking to themselves but wanting you to hear it as a witness.

A sense of achievement

A sense of achievement can also provide supportive meaning to a person. Benedict, a counsellor, told the story of Monica, a mature student, who was looking for support to see her through her last year in university.

> *Monica had been seriously ill and was declared cancer free, yet she looked as if she was in her sixties, not her forties. Her marriage had collapsed and she said 'I am not a woman anymore, just a carcass walking around'. She was frightened that on top of being physically damaged by surgery, she would turn out to be an intellectual failure as well. Benedict was determined to try and help her get her degree. They concentrated on learning the skills of how to study effectively and as Monica's academic work gave evidence of her intelligence, she began to feel more of a person again. She ended her counselling with a kiss saying 'Thank you Benedict, you have done the trick'.*

He explained:

> *Monica had rediscovered an ability to relate. It was almost as if she knew that it would be acceptable for her to come over and kiss me and I wasn't going to experience her as a kind of wizened, dried out, totally inhuman kind of carcass. I have no idea what she meant by saying 'You've done the trick', but what I heard from it was that I had enabled her to do the only thing left worthwhile for her to accomplish; that is to get her degree, and thus discover some self-valuation.*

When she came into counselling, Monica had lost her sense of self. Her illness, the marriage break-up that ensued, and her difficulty in completing the studies she had chosen to take up in mid-life made her look down on herself as an 'inhuman kind of carcass'. One can assume that she may have seen this judgement reflected in the eyes of people she came across. Even her therapist mentioned she looked awful, with a very white, wizened face. With her academic success, Monica rediscovered her self-respect and with it another way of being. Pleased with what she had accomplished, she regained the ability to relate and the meaning this gave to her life was healing and restorative.

Arthur, whom we met in the previous chapter, had also become estranged from his family. He too discovered during his illness another way of being himself and relating to others. This was uplifting for him and transforming for him and his family.

Recognising one's identity and status

An important issue of identity when we think about death is that, as individuals, it is commonly very difficult for us to imagine what it will be like for the world to go on without us. A client had a large photograph above the mantelpiece, showing all her family, minus the youngest grandson, who was born after the photograph was taken. When this little one was old enough to recognise his family in the photograph he could not understand why he was not there. Even at a young age we start to think about our identity and where we fit in.

As we previously noted, Rebecca, a patient in the hospice where Alice works as a chaplain, surprised everybody by getting to her son's wedding and not even sitting in most of the photographs. Alice continued:

> After the wedding, Rebecca bargained again. She wanted to be there for her other son's birthday and later again was determined that she hadn't finished all the things that she wanted to do as a teacher. Rebecca almost forced herself up again. She was struggling so hard to keep alive. This had become almost pathological. Because she didn't want to lose control, she was becoming more and more controlling of everybody else around her, which was very hard for her family.

Rebecca's sense of self was adrift. At one point she said 'I have things I want to do as a teacher', by which she meant 'I am a teacher, but actually at the moment I cannot be, so who am I?' And maybe 'I am a wife, I am a mother, but at the moment I cannot be, so who am I?' 'I have not finished my role and nobody can look after my house like me, so who am I?' Rebecca felt that she had a role to fulfil as a mother at her son's wedding. But her story shows a bigger picture: her controlling strength of mind and determination was hard on her relatives and carers. In her fight to survive, she was trying to tell them: 'Without me you are lost'. This delayed the family's opportunity to say their goodbyes. Determination can sometimes become aggression and that can leave the family in further confusion.

A number of restrictions and limitations often come with illness. Patients stop working, they cannot do their usual jobs in and outside the home, nor can they continue to fulfil their role in the community. Eventually they become more and more dependent on the care of others. Eve referred to her client Susan, who found it very difficult to adjust to not being the carer she used to be. She continued the struggle to come to terms with her sense of self and, in Eve's perception, had a difficult ending.

> *Susan was a vicar's wife and she'd been very involved in the parish until she developed multiple sclerosis and physically went downhill very quickly. In the family, too, Susan used to be the one in charge. She made things happen. She was the motivator behind her husband Jim, who suffered from dementia. He worried about her when they were separated due to her long hospital stays, but he appeared to be quite content with it. When their son brought Jim in to see her, he would sit in the wheelchair and just smile. Susan could see that he was almost untroubled and well cared for, but she found that difficult to accept.*
>
> *Susan had two sons. The one who came in every day to see her had been in trouble in various ways. He was a bit of a disgrace, which had been difficult for a public figure like a vicar. The other son ignored her almost completely during her illness but, married with two daughters, he was the model son in society. Susan felt great anger. If her son and family did visit, she tended to be cross with them. Maybe that's why they kept away. Yet she would say, 'I'm so lucky, I'm so lucky,' almost aggressively.*
>
> *What Susan said more than anything else was, 'I must battle on. I must get well'. She had always been the one to help others, support her husband, look after the sons, help her friends, be there and do practical things. She could not let go of that. Eventually, her body just gave out. She couldn't fight anymore. She had a slow death; not particularly painful, but which made her incredibly weary. It was hard for her.*

Susan could not settle down with changing her self-image. She had been relied on to do things, and she could not let go of that perceived responsibility. Because of her limiting illness, she had lost that caring part of herself, and without it she could not see who she was. Susan fought all the way and was unhappy. Yet she felt that she ought to be thankful, and so repeated almost in that aggressive way 'I'm so lucky'. It was Susan's resistance to change which contributed to her difficult ending. In contrast, another patient, Luke, had a more positive attitude, which Eve believed made for a good death, even though it was very uncomfortable physically.

> *Luke was an alcoholic. He'd been admitted to hospital a lot. He held down a job until retirement, but alcohol had been a part of his life since youth. It had been for his father too. Luke's mother doted on him. She wouldn't believe that he was an alcoholic, which was hard for his sister and brother because he was the ne'er-do-well and they were the responsible ones. Mother had leant on Luke as her marriage broke up, building him up to expectations he couldn't fulfil and he had turned to drink very early on.*
>
> *When I met Luke he'd been told that he wouldn't recover. How long he lived depended on whether he drank or not. They talked about liver transplants, but he didn't want to go through that. His life had reached fulfilment. He was very kind to his sister and brother and they to him as he was quite demanding with all his hospital admissions. He found great satisfaction that he'd been loved by them. He had organised everything; not that he had huge wealth, but every-thing he had would be for them and their children.*
>
> *Luke used to hold my hand as I prayed. I knew somehow that he was ready to go. His faith was very much part of him, but he didn't articulate it. At the funeral it became clear how he had supported other people and made friends. But it wasn't his reason for being, so when he couldn't be a good friend any more it was enough that he was just him, loved by his sister and brother and, he believed, accepted by God. He was ready to let go, and being poorly had some part in that. Perhaps he had had enough of struggling.*

Somehow Luke had reached contentment with his life. Even though Eve could not say he had 'a good life' by usual standards, he was able to remember what was good in his. The fact that he was loved by God was planted within him, in some ways at a more profound level than for Susan, who lived more in the perspective of 'what you do is important' and 'you must be good'. Susan had been 'good', Luke had not, but somehow for him it was enough simply to be. This made it easier for him and for his family towards the end because they had a very calm, peaceful accepting person to be with. Susan made this shift too, but only very near the end when her body gave out and she could fight no longer.

Susan and Luke's stories draw attention to how the patient's acceptance of real situations can foster honest, open, and meaningful communication, which is sustaining. They also help us to acknowledge the important role of the dying body in the process of surrender. Eve shares her thoughts:

> The body is kind to us when it gets tired and weary because patients think they could leave this body behind and that probably helps. It helped Luke to know that he was dying. It almost carried him. His family felt that he had made peace with himself and with God. His faith rose with the illness and he was able to talk to them about dying and about what he would like for his funeral.

It is a very moving mystery how body, mind, and spirit interact when death draws near. One of us was touched to witness this process in a lady who was living her last months. She was of a considerable age and part of her was weary of life, but another part was very anxious about dying and this was revealed in delusions and agitation. As she got weaker and her bodily functions increasingly gave up, something shifted. She started recognising and accepting that she would not get better and that she was on her last journey. Between periods of sleep she became more present and one day, about a month before she died, she said: *'There's a lot of work going on in here'* pointing to her chest. The weakening of her body helped to ease her mind and enabled her to deal with issues of life and death, reviewing what had been and accepting what was ahead.

References

Gould, P. 2012. *When I Die. Lessons from the Death Zone*. London: Atom, an imprint of Little, Brown.

Frankl, V. 2004. *Man's Search for Meaning*. London: Rider.

Jung, C. G. 1992. *Psychological Types*. London: Routledge.

Part 2

The impact on family carers

Chapter 5

Demands on the family

Many jobs in life are demanding on the worker's time, skills, and energies. Most are applied for; the demands are accepted as part of the package and are likely to be reflected in the salary or wages involved. The role and job of a family carer is usually set within a very different framework. It is not applied for; the demands can be enormous and can quickly change, at times becoming total. There is, far from financial gain, the probability of financial loss. The role is imposed because of family or marital bonds, frequently without regard for the skills and experience acquired. It is often for the long term, within changing circumstances.

This brief résumé describes the framework of the lives of hundreds of thousands of people in the UK who care for someone suffering life-limiting or life-threatening illness. It is truly a call for duty, which in the case of the carer as well as the patient, can be life-altering, and carries little recognition amongst most outside and non-participating observers. It is these heroes and heroines we consider in this chapter.

As in the previous chapters, we will take into consideration the social, psychological, and moral demands on people and their support networks. We will also recognise and take account of the impact of the community in which the family lives and the financial and intervention policies of the welfare state. These important matters, vital as they are, will be treated as powerful backdrops to our main focus of how individual people cope with the challenging and stressful circumstances that are laid on carers by the major illness of another person in the home or family circle, and where and how they look for healing and support.

While we concentrate on carers who are family members or friends, it must not be forgotten that there are also professionals and other volunteers coming into the home to offer assistance: nurses, live-in and visiting carers, community nurse specialists, physiotherapists, and others who are employed by the local authority, care organisations, charities like MacMillan and Marie Curie, or the local hospice. Their contribution, which is considered in depth in Part 3, is considerable, but it is limited in time and role definition. It is the family carer who lives with the problem all the time, and this brings its own strains and insights. Life-altering illness puts the whole family under a considerable amount of stress.

Diagnosis and its demands

The role of the family or friend carer is rarely planned for. It comes out of the blue, virtually without warning, for even if early symptoms are indicated, they are frequently misunderstood or ignored. It is at diagnosis that the truth is revealed. A threatening diagnosis for cancer, a chronic heart condition, or a neurological disease can turn the life of the patient and their family upside down. Things are not going to be the same. Well-trodden paths of attitude, outlook, roles, custom, expectation, and hopes will all be changed. The husband, wife or partner, son or daughter in a matter of minutes becomes a patient; their partners, parents, and friends, become carers, supporters, encouragers, perhaps even the breadwinner. It is a harrowing and threatening situation for most, replete with loss, risk, uncertainty, and questioning.

Leslie tells a vivid story of when his wife was diagnosed with cancer, which highlights many of the facets associated with such times.

Following a consultation and tests, my wife and I were invited to go to the hospital to talk things over with the consultant. We were shown into a small room where there were three doctors including the consultant sitting behind a desk. The consultant welcomed us in a friendly way, then his face changed and he told us that the news was bad. Anna had a nasty form of cancer, which he and his colleagues would have to investigate further and quickly. 'I am very sorry' he said and he then got up with his two colleagues and as he was leaving the room, he told us that one of his colleagues would be back in a few minutes.

We just looked at one another—we were both stunned, and Anna started to cry. 'Am I going to die? What are they going to do to me?' she asked. I felt sick. I did not know what to say. I put my arms round her and felt like crying myself. In a few minutes, one of the doctors came back and asked if he could come in. 'It is going to be a tough journey, but we will be strongly on your side' he said. 'We must now look to see if the cancer has spread and to work out what we must do.' He opened a sheaf of paper and told my wife that she would be admitted immediately. He then asked me to go home and fetch a bag of personal things for Anna. 'We will make a plan as soon as we have the information we need. Then we will get under way. The sooner the better.'

The doctor clearly thought that haste would be an encouragement to us. It was quite the opposite; the seriousness of Anna's situation and mine was being confirmed. After a few more questions, he told us that a nurse would come back in a short time to take Anna to a ward. He then left. Once again we were on our own, torn apart, but clinging to one another. I felt helpless, hopeless. Anna looked desperate and fearful. A nurse arrived and took her away. I left and drove home to get a bag of things. Quite the most awful day of my life! I felt devastated and alone. I could not imagine what Anna felt in that huge, strange place.

Leslie and Anna had no idea what was to happen. They felt unable to ask questions. They were not given much opportunity to do so. At one level, the doctors were kindly. They clearly felt for the couple, but their professional boundary was associated with getting on with things in pursuit of a cure, or at least a diminution of the damage. Speed was of the essence; little attention was paid to the impact on Leslie and Anna or the giving to them of any personal support or encouragement. For them the impact was devastating, partly out of fear at the extent of the unknown and unspecified medical issue, partly out of a sense of not knowing what would be the consequences, and partly the sudden and unexpected, even short, separation that was involved while the further investigations were under way. Leslie returned home to a 'quiet, dead house which was no longer sunny but cold and strange'.

That 'most awful day of his life' gave Leslie a sense of world change. Not only had the house and home changed in his eyes, but his whole environment became full of dark clouds instead of sunshine. The patient and her husband shared the impact of the news, but only one became the primary focus of interest. The other, the carer, had to stand back and be supportive, sensitive to the other's needs, positive and active, however much he felt to the contrary. Grief as to what could be lost in the life not lived would be mutual, even if not identical, and only one of them would really be free to express it. The suddenness of the news left no room for preparation, adjustment, or planning, even if in retrospect it was not a total surprise, as signs of failing health were recalled but which at the time had been minimised or ignored.

One of the dominant factors emerging from Leslie's story is the importance of accurate, carefully expressed information. The couple's fear was aroused by ignorance of what was to be, what the priorities would mean. Ignorance exacerbated their fear and their sense of helplessness as against the professional confidence of the doctors. Once Leslie had had an open and trusting discussion with his GP, he was able to pull himself together. The issues and dangers had not changed, but his attitude towards them became more resolute. Shock and fear may be inevitable in the circumstances, but they can be managed to become proportionate to the illness. With a gradual coping with the news can come a review of the practical matters involved, such as where help can be obtained, or what are the financial implications. Sometimes, unresolved conflicts need to be sorted out and, if possible, wrongs or mistakes corrected. Some of the debris of the past needs to be dropped, as a new challenging life begins and searching questions addressed: 'How serious?', 'How long?', 'Where will it end?', 'What path will have to be taken?'

Another carer, Jack, talked to us:

> *The shock at diagnosis was devastating but then my confidence increased as my partner's illness was very slow to develop. This raised my hopes that a mistake had been made. But gradually the tingling in the fingers indicative of multiple sclerosis became a numbness and lack of coordination. My spirits dropped. I began to share the experience of the rollercoaster so common in neurological diseases. Now my partner's condition oscillates between significant developments and remissions. 'I sometimes don't know what to think'.*

The ups and downs of the rollercoaster, which can go on for years, leave the carer, let alone the patient, with a sense of no settled outlook. Variations can literally be by the day; there is no room for the confidence arising from familiarity. The constant uncertainty can bring inner tensions and the consequences of a restlessness and sense of oppression. One of our informants, Howard, told us:

> *Such was my difficulty with rapid variation and changes that I began to wonder who was the patient: 'My settled life was a wreck, and I could not blame anyone except God'. My longing for some form of certainty, however grim, became a constant facet, but one that presented no solution.*

We are reminded that the 'longing for normality and yearning for safety' is applicable to both patients and carers.

Logistics

In other chapters we note the sense of dependency of patients and carers on the medical profession, the hospitals and the courses of treatment undertaken. This frequently leads to an indisputable priority of getting to treatment over all other factors. It becomes the absolute dominant issue. The household routines are adapted, transport arrangements, however complicated. are undertaken.

> *One of the carers we consulted, Joyce, drove her husband over 50 miles each way every day for five weeks, leaving each morning at 6 am. The stresses and strains on patient and carer must have been considerable, but the programme was completed; at what cost physically, psychologically, and indeed financially can only be imagined.*

Such stresses are often compounded by having to accommodate changed appointment dates and times, inconveniencing school and work commitments.

Logistics do not only involve travel. A number of our carer reporters told us of how responsibility, sometimes total, was passed to them by their ill spouse. New tasks, such as managing the finances, had to be taken up for the first time and, in the case of some male carers, they had to learn basic cooking, to organise the domestic arrangements, and to come to terms with the skills of intimate caring of another person. The rhythm of an early life and its routines disappeared and were replaced by uncertainty, confusion, and often loneliness.

Logistical issues can be compounded by the circumstances in which the caring is taking place. The house may be small with many steps and narrow doors. The bathroom may be unsuitable for use by a weak or disabled person. Hospital beds may be needed and appropriately positioned downstairs—no small matter in modest-sized houses, and a severe disruption to the home. Domestic houses are not built for long-term patients and these changes can be awkward and add considerably to the carer's burden. The local authority or charity may be able to provide vital assistance with handrails, chairlifts, and bath adaptations, but the general inconvenience remains.

Another common factor for the carer is that there may be other members of the family resident, especially when the patient is younger. This part of the family will also need attention to their physical and emotional needs. For instance, children must be fed, delivered to school, supervised and supported.

> One of our informants, June, had a partner who had longstanding Parkinson's disease. But also within her household she had to care for her own elderly mother as well as her daughter and her disturbed son. We wondered at her courage and capacity, for in addition to this domestic scene, she also worked full time.

Carers often have need of superhuman energy and liberal doses of adrenaline, but June points to a limitation far beyond that which should be expected of any one person. When asked about that, she accepted that there was no realistic alternative, although another family member enabled her to take occasional short breaks. We still wondered at her capacity and grit, but feared for her long-term well-being. Her hyper-activity was based on the conviction that it was her duty and that if she failed to fulfil it she would feel profoundly guilty.

Finance

For many families, especially the less affluent, the struggle for finance is very important. Costs, visible and hidden, often rise along with the severity of the illness. Among many other costs, transport, parking, keeping the house warmer, or paying for some domestic help, make considerable demands on the budget. These expenses often arise at the same time as income is being seriously eroded or even lost. The patient may no longer be able to work and the carer is forced to cut their working hours to attend clinic appointments and to look after the patient.

Medical support for the sick and disabled can be enormous, due to the National Health Service and its fundamental concept of services being free at the point of delivery. The State is not so generous when it comes to social and domestic support. While grants and benefits are generally pitched more favourably towards the less well-off, they do not solve the problem. In recent history, legislation has limited benefits to what might be considered to be provision for minimum standards. The various allowances and benefits are often complicated to understand and are frequently means-tested or dependent on National Insurance contributions. Lay people may well need to seek professional guidance from bodies such as the Citizen's Advice Bureau, Social Services, or MacMillan information centres, so as to make the fullest use of such funds. These may come towards either supporting the patient financially or providing regular and consistent care. Nevertheless, considerable reliance still has to be placed on private or family assets and funds over the long term. Even with this support there is therefore a strong likelihood that, alongside all the other stresses, finance becomes a major problem for many families.

Teamwork

In her commitment to the care of her husband, June brought forward a number of important issues. We have already pointed out that caring involves a whole range of requirements that must be managed carefully. No one person can or should do everything. Stress and exhaustion can soon arise. The situation is not helped by the common factor that there is at times no obvious assistance to hand, and that it could be felt to be awkward or embarrassing to ask for it. It is common that carers feel unique in being the only person who would be acceptable to the patient or can handle the routines. Family carers can become isolated from their circle of friends because of the care demands upon them. These can often start quite modestly, but as the disease develops, they can become all-embracing and oppressive. Research has shown that patients' distress is at its highest at the time of first diagnosis and recurrence (Silberfarb *et al.*, 1980), but for the family the palliative and terminal phases of illness on the other hand prove particularly demanding (Cassileth *et al.*, 1985). Carer isolation can lead to this sense of loneliness, and loneliness to depression and a profound sense of loss; not only of friends and family, but of life as it was once known.

The tragedy is that often the level of commitment of carers and their sense of being essential is not positive or even necessary. If other people can be involved in the care, and the family carer can see herself as the leader of a team, then their outlook is much brighter, as indeed is that of the patient. There is the potential for a sense of corporate warmth, a variety of approach to the work, and mutual support, which all contribute to a more effective sustaining of the standard of care. To seek help is not a sign of weakness but a sign of strength. A realisation of needs and personal limitations can lead to positive reappraisal and effective results for patient and carer. Help need not come only from volunteers and friends but can be available through the local medical and social support structures. A discussion with the GP or community nurse can be a valuable starter.

While the above suggestions are positive, we have found amongst our informants that their personal sense of duty and the anxiety about leaving 'their' patient can override seeking or accepting help. The basis of such a sense of duty can be a commitment to the marriage vows 'in sickness and in health', a feeling that care is owed as a payback for earlier support and generosity by the patient, or a sense of guilt for a past or present failing. These factors are real and powerful, but they can be damaging to balanced decisions and can in turn place the carer under the risk of breakdown. The practical response is not always proportionate and rational when it comes to reacting to the call of loyalty or faithfulness, to the wedding vows, to love and care in all circumstances, or from a sense of thanksgiving for what has been previously received. It is vital for good long-term care that there is cooperation and respect between carers, including outside professionals and members of the family or circle of friends who are willing and able to help. It is also important that there is awareness of one's own limitations.

Assistance from family and friends is available more frequently than is perhaps recognised. Their failure to offer help is often due to a fear of interfering or intruding or being refused. On the other hand, it is also true that people like to be asked to help. It brings recognition of their importance and value as friends or neighbours and of the skills that they may have to offer. There may well be limitations necessary, but people are often willing to assist as far as is possible.

The other substantial source of help is that by professional carers. However, problems can arise between the lay carer and visiting professionals when their respective functions are misunderstood. Family carers can be resentful at one extreme and overdependent and with excessive expectations on another. Therefore, appreciation of the function of both professionals and family carers is necessary. Family carers know the patient very well; a trust and understanding could have been built up over decades and so they can become excessively identified with the patient and his illness. It is difficult for them to be both empathetic and objective. They can be anxious, short-tempered, and forceful with members of the professional services, and even with the patient: sadly patients are sometimes abused. The family carer's situation, one without escape, must be recognised by the professionals when they visit. They must be tolerant and patient. At times the family carer can become the client.

We generally assume that family carers have known the patient a long time, but this is not always the case. As people live longer, new relationships are forged long after people in previous generations would have died. We see today people in their sixties, seventies, and even eighties bonding together in new marriages or partnerships. When one of the parties becomes ill, they cannot fall back on the long process of growing together. The depth of companionship can be threatened and it can bring extra doubts and stresses on the new partner, who is unexpectedly called upon to care for the other. This also brings particular disappointments or frustrations, and occasionally resentment to the carer's family. A new relationship between older people brings joys and new life, but it can also be, and is likely to be, shorter lived. The consequences of this fact are not always appreciated at the outset by the couple concerned, or by their families, who may resent the cost of caring for (or indeed sharing inheritance with) someone who is not a blood relation.

The vast majority of family carers are mature adults; indeed many are elderly and infirm themselves, but there is a significant proportion of patients being cared for by young adults, and even children. One of us knew until recently a girl of 12, looking after her mother who was bedridden with ME (chronic fatigue syndrome).

> *Katie attended school, so she had to fulfil many of the carer tasks before she went and to prepare the main meal on her return. She is a courageous and resourceful person, but one who is in danger of being deprived of a normal upbringing through the circumstances. Her mother did all she could to assist, but at times that was very limited. Katie had to respond and did so with commitment and with the professional assistance which came to the house during the day. Nevertheless, Katie missed out on many of the experiences and indeed fun of her peers.*

Older children also, young adults themselves, often with families and responsibility of work, can find the additional pressures of tending a seriously ill parent or sibling very demanding. This can impose strain on their own relationships and working patterns.

When recognition does exist, good relationships may develop, to the benefit of patient and carer. It is in the interest and policy of the social and the health authorities to keep people at home, if at all possible and appropriate, rather than in hospital or in a nursing home. This policy is also the popular wish of most patients and families, but it can put great strains on local resources. A network of nurses, physiotherapists, counsellors, and other advisors is available and can be called upon by general practitioners. There are occasional costs arising, but many of the services are free. Whilst such professional callers to the home may come and go, they bring their skilled help and advice to the carer and the patient and offer them personal support and friendship. Further help and facilities are also available from the local hospice. Nevertheless, demand is growing fast and resources are limited. No doubt a challenge to creativity lies ahead in finding new ways of meeting the growing demands while honouring the holistic approach of the hospice ideal and the contributions of many other services within the community.

References

Cassileth, B. R., Lusk, E. J. and Strouse, T. B. 1985. A psychological analysis of cancer patients and their next-of-kin. *Cancer*, **55**, 72–76.

Silberfarb, P. M., Maurer, L. H. and Crouthamel, C. S. 1980. Psychosocial aspects of neoplastic disease: 1. Functional status of breast cancer patients during different treatment regimes. *American Journal of Psychiatry*, **137**, 450–455.

Chapter 6

Lives taken over

Cancer has
Hijacked my body.
Ensnared my soul.
My world has become smaller,
Orbiting around chemo cycles, hospital visits and my bed.
Time has an altered rhythm,
Hours go by more slowly.
Every day brings a new challenge—but some days a
Robin's wordless song transports me,
Another day the sun might shine through my bedroom window.
Pleasure has been distilled.
Yes, each new day offers a pure gift.

Ger Byrne, reproduced with kind permission of the author.

When illness strikes in a reasonably settled life, there is no time to prepare and it can take over all of one's life. With time to think about it, images of surgery, discomfort, and helplessness, invade the mind. After a first moment of total distress and being shattered, a number of patients and carers move on to ask 'Why me?' and to express the anxiety and anger involved in that.

We have seen patient reactions along the line of: 'Well, if I'm going to die, I might as well give up now. It's too painful almost to go on living, so I'm just going to close down'. These can be the hardest patients for carers to be alongside. There seems to be no glimmer of light and this can lead to a dragging down of the whole family. This in turn may provoke a sense of failure on their part because they think that they do not have enough to make a significant difference to the well-being of the patient.

Conversely, for some patients, there may come a point of looking back at 'What have I done with my life?' There may also be that moment when suddenly they know they are going to die and that somehow shifts their attention towards asking 'What am I going to do with the time that I have left?' A number of them get to grips with the fact that they have a choice about how they spend their remaining time. Such choices can radically change their experience of it. Even if constrained by their physical limitations and all sorts of other reasons, one of which is the technical competence and knowledge of the medical profession on whom one feels properly reliant, patients still have choice and control, sometimes over very tiny things, but that is still important. These choices are likely to affect others.

Changing experience of time

The experience of the passage of time and people's relation to it can become an important issue in life-threatening illness. Patients react in very personal ways to illness and all they have to work through. What is supportive for one may be abhorred by another. Some people are prepared to try almost anything to experience the hope of keeping the inevitable at bay. They are in a sense buying time. For others, looking ahead and making arrangements for and beyond their death is top priority; they do not want to talk about the past. New hurdles need to be worked on and perhaps in a particular order. The things that become easier to do are often the practical things, like deciding on their funeral arrangements, making the wills, and sorting out financial matters or making sure that the partner knows how to use the washing machine! What sometimes gets overlooked, for which there seems not enough energy or time available, are the relational things: whether there is anything they need to do with someone. Reassured and feeling good about themselves by doing the practical things, patients, their family, and carers may tend to postpone the far less predictable and more challenging being in relationship.

The mental states of both patient and carer affect and are affected by their experience of time, leading sometimes to discouragement or the sense of being on a rollercoaster of hopes and setbacks. Time and its demands, heightened by uncertainty and dread of 'something', becomes the frame for mixed and confused feelings.

> *We remember a lady so thankful for her husband's remission that she wanted to believe in a miracle. When the time came for all treatment to be stopped she was completely devastated; she could not or would not believe the situation had changed in such a radical way. For the patient on the other hand, the medical decision to stop treatment meant the very end was only a stone throw away; death became his overriding concern: for her, it was the thinking about her loss and future life. This very challenging situation for both of them was compounded by the clash in their experience and perspective and the resultant difficulty in talking and being with each other.*

Mismatching of individual perceptions can feel disruptive and even disrespectful at times. It may be hard to try to understand or comprehend each other's point of view and isolation, loneliness, and missed opportunities can ensue.

Not only are there different perceptions of time and their significance, but also an understanding of time itself. What does 'urgent' mean? How important is 'urgent'? Does it mean immediate action? Sometimes 'urgent' cases are delayed for months. These questions are made real as we recall the doctor's reaction to Anna's diagnosis, which required immediate action (see Chapter 5, 'Diagnosis and its demands'). The doctor saw immediate action as a curative necessity, but Anna and Leslie took it as a great threat and an underpinning of their fear of what was to happen. However the speed of response can also be seen as a message of hope. Philip Gould suggests that the speed of medical response made his diagnosis bearable for him 'creating a sense of struggle, purpose and endpoint' (Gould, 2012 p. 45). All are struggling in their own way with hope, despair, and angst, but probably also with the feeling that everything seems to be on pause while waiting for unpredictable test results. Discrepancies can easily happen between patient and carers, particularly doctors. Time can feel like eternity for those likely to receive bad news, while for those who are busy time can appear to pass in a flash.

Time may be an agent of healing or the purveyor of new threat. Expectations change as the illness continues. Immediately post-surgery, pain and scars tend to dominate the mind. The further some get away from disease and treatment, the more confidence they have that they will recover. For others, expectations become adapted and perhaps more modest. As Billy put it:

> There is a transition from hope that you'll get better to hope that you'll be able to get in a wheelchair in the garden, or achieve someone's wedding or just have a day free of symptoms.

Being discharged from hospital or treatment holds its own challenges, such as facing up to having a future and managing ordinary life without the support that was so readily available during the critical phase of the illness.

When patients and carers are in the thrall of transition and change, the numbers on the dial of a clock may seem to gain or lose their importance. Patients may feel in a sort of 'time-out'; life is on hold. In such times, the *quality* of the present moment (*Καιρος—kairos*) can take precedence over its *duration* (*Χρόνος—chronos*). *Chronos* is time in terms of a clock. The tick of every second records its passing. On the other hand, *kairos* is about what that *chronos* means, its quality and impact. *Kairos* can provide opportunities for a response—it can mark out a future and produce a change: perhaps it becomes 'a moment of truth'—while *chronos* is inexorable. Philip Gould is drawing out this distinction when he writes:

> All of us tend to think in terms of linear time. One thing follows another. But this is only one form of time's many complexities. I can no longer think like that. What good is it to me to think in terms of conventional time? Six months or nine months no longer exist for me. So I am trying to make sense of the world not through time but through emotion, through relationships, through feeling. (Gould, 2012 p. 134)

As Gould says, emotions, relationships, and feelings may become increasingly important while at the same time practical issues appear to take precedence.

The understanding and the experience of time will have implications for the therapy. For instance, in the light of a patient's prognosis, there may not be enough time to address personal issues of depression and anxiety in depth. Encouraging communication and understanding in the family becomes more important. In addition, when their end draws near, patients do not have the strength for long conversations, and counselling encounters tend to be shorter and more frequent.

For patients and those around the bedside, variations in their awareness of time and their expectations can be felt in a range of senses such as rhythm, urgency, patience, fullness, emptiness, boredom, and connectedness among others. We could describe this with a metaphor: doctors are on the motorways to diagnosis, treatment, and results; families and friends are on a rollercoaster of fast and slow traffic and do not always enjoy the journey. Patients travel the winding country lanes, discovering the unknown around every bend, learning along the way, bored, frustrated, or enthused by what they meet. Moreover, family and care team juggle different timescales: of jobs, shopping, illness, running the household, and the like. On the other hand the patient may tend to feel locked in a maze where all the roads run towards or around him and his illness, comfort, prospects, feelings, and expectations. Michael Mayne (2006) vividly described how his world contracted. His concerns centred around the illness and his body changes. His sleep was affected by the anticipation and anxiety that crept up on him in the dark hours of the night. Such feelings made him more self-centred and aware and, he tells us, 'self-concern is a near neighbour of self-indulgence'. (Mayne, 2006 p. XIX)

Carers, professionals, friends, and family can be tempted to minimise or deny the contraction of the patient's world. In order to overcome this they may focus on fostering a sense of inner peace and/or filling the day with activities and complementary therapies, which may be new and exciting for the patient but also potentially exhausting. Readers who are familiar with bereavement support may recognise something of this when they help a person understand that the door to the beloved has been shut and will not be reopened, at least in this world. Another door may open, but dismissing the reality of the loss is a fraud, tempting as this may be sometimes for the carer who tries to comfort. The beloved has gone, whether or not new doors open. The temptation to soften this difficult reality is potent, but sooner or later it needs to be dealt with, and often carers can help more by doing so with empathy and loving attention than by minimising the loss.

Priorities and decision making

In the light of the limited time available to both patients and carers, priorities can change. Things that seemed important can become trivial and other things that people hardly noticed before suddenly move to centre-stage. Wanting to do things while they still can, patients need to negotiate choices involving family and loved ones, and they may run the risk of becoming out of step with each other. Being attentive to everyone's needs is a fine balancing act, especially during a medical crisis with its various demands.

When Jennifer, one of our informants was herself recalled after a mammogram, she went through the suspense of waiting for diagnosis and was surprised at what surfaced:

> It was a huge relief to be told that there was no growth. During the week that I had to think about the possibility and the treatment, I was swinging between 'yes I do' and 'no I don't' go for treatment. I thought about the horror of having the surgery, the whole assault on my body and the revulsion of going through the chemo, the cutting up.
>
> On the other hand, I thought that having cancer would help me prioritise my life. I did not share that with anyone but I imagined that being bereft of the perspective of 'having time' would make me put my house in order and simplify my life. It would be an opportunity to focus on unfinished business. That was the thought, aside from all the fear and the revulsion, and that was in a way consoling.
>
> But I realise that I may not have felt the same had I not done this work and heard women say 'I feel more sorted', 'I know it's important to me that I have left my job', 'I used to let that bother me, and now that seems trivial'.

When life becomes time-limited, people can become impatient with or intolerant of another's problems. Personal things that take up time and energy can be seen in a new light. Some patients and carers talk about installing 'me-time'. Whilst they would have felt guilty about lying down, having a rest in the afternoon, or doing something for pleasure or fulfilment, they have learned to spend money and time on themselves.

When the illness becomes critical, there can be a shift in priorities, not only in what becomes a priority, but the order in which they are tackled. Alice, a chaplain, comments:

I see it with a lot of people. It is not just one thing that needs to be dealt with, it is a whole series. It is like a show-jumping ring. You know if you take your horse into the ring, you have to go over all the jumps, but there's a particular order. You need to have all your concentration on jump number one, until you are over that and then all your concentration on number two. You are vaguely aware of the rest of the course, but you concentrate on one hurdle at a time.

People with a life-altering illness may find themselves having to make difficult decisions as they face different hurdles, such as their sense of how they are, their job, their financial situation, the children, the husband, the wider family and social network, as well as their health, symptoms, pain, anger, and anxiety. As Alice suggests, some resolution may allow the next issue to be dealt with, but there is not always enough time for hoped for or planned decisions to work out.

We remember Janet, a patient whose husband had to organise a move to a level bungalow for her to come home in a wheelchair. The children were terrified at the prospect of moving and leaving their friends and neighbourhood. It was poignant to think of that man having to deal with organising his wife's return home, knowing that she may not be around for much longer, and in doing so taking the children out of a supportive neighbourhood they were going to need in the coming months and years. Major decisions were made to fit Janet's needs, giving her hope and perspective. She spent one afternoon in the new home before dying in the hospice.

This poignant story highlights how the priorities, demands, and desires can differ for the people involved. The children quite understandably did not want to leave their friends and familiar neighbourhood even though they were yearning for their mother to come home. The husband, together with Janet or on his own, spent a lot of energy and time negotiating with estate agents and builders to organise a fitting place for his spouse to come home to. The associated stresses and concerns deprived them of precious quality time together and with the children, and all too soon Janet's husband and children were facing a double bereavement: for Janet and for the loss of their familiar home. This story also demonstrates for us how terminal illness can produce a framework of time for any decision. The more serious the illness, the more emphatic the framework. Not only does it limit the scope of what is framed, but it also sharpens the issue concerned and the other priorities that might replace it.

The struggle over priorities can be about practical jobs and tasks to be ful-filled; it can also be connected to the character of the people involved and how it impacts on their relationships. We are reminded here of the loss of status experienced by Susan, the highly involved vicar's wife who could not let go of being the one in charge (see Chapter 4, 'Recognising one's identity and sta-tus'), and Rebecca, the teacher who wanted to be at her son's wedding and made it against all odds (see Chapter 2, 'Some personal sources of strength' and Chapter 4, 'Recognising one's identity and status'). For both these patients, their family's admiration for their loved one's determination and courage to 'manage' went hand in hand with the loss of an opportunity to prepare for a future without them or to share a peaceful ending with them.

The reality of unpredictability

No one knows the course of an illness in detail. Estimates of remaining life-times are only probabilities, not certainties. The not knowing can undermine attempts to make life plans, after treatment as well as when undergoing it.

For some people a sense of knowing can be very important. They organise their life and rearrange their priorities accordingly.

> We remember a patient who had been told that she had three months to live. When she exceeded that time, she became extremely angry and upset. She had taken the doctor's word for certainty and felt cheated. Setting her mind on making the most of her remaining time, she travelled as much as she could and gave away her estate. Unexpectedly alive beyond the estimated time frame, she had to face up to financial and other worries that she had not counted on and which could have been avoided.

Planning ahead and knowing what to expect allows us to be prepared, and some people derive a sense of security from that while others are harassed or stressed by that knowledge. Rachel, a counsellor who led groups for women with breast cancer secondaries tells the story of Olivia:

> Olivia was very open about what she was living with. She would talk about feeling that the end was coming and shared how she wanted her funeral to be organised. She was an atheist who cared for the environment and had it all worked out. She talked in a very humorous way in the group about what she did and did not want. A few mouths fell open, but she carried on.
>
> I remember the last time Olivia came, she felt obviously ill and she was a bit in a panic when she felt she couldn't talk properly. I just sat with her and in the last half hour she found her voice, her breathing improved and she was able to talk, very deeply again, about where she was and her wishes for the family. She

really wanted to live until her youngest son was through his exams at university. She died a month later in the hospice and I am so sad that she didn't make it till her son's graduation.

Olivia had it all worked out and could talk about her death and funeral openly. Sadly, her life could not finish the way she had hoped. She failed to attend her son's graduation.

In both these examples we see patients making plans and wishes they hoped to be able to fulfil. This reminds us of how important it can be for patients to make sense of their experience and find meaning. Discovering this, even if it is a negative understanding, reduces the threat of unpredictability, which for some is hardly bearable. Carers will be well advised to keep this in mind when talking to patients about what they are led to expect. This may help them to be careful not to give false hope or raise undue fears. In the end, everyone of us needs to remember that we all live unpredictable lives.

Acknowledgements

Text extracts from Gould, P., *When I die: Lessons from the death zone*, Atom, an imprint of Little, Brown Book Group, London, UK, Copyright © 2012, reproduced with permission from Little, Brown Book Group.

Text extracts from Mayne, M., *The Enduring Melody*, Darton, Longman and Todd, London, UK, Copyright © 2006, reproduced with permission from Darton, Longman and Todd publishers.

References

Gould, P. 2012. *When I Die. Lessons from the Death Zone.* London: Atom, an imprint of Little, Brown.

Mayne, M. 2006. *The Enduring Melody*, London: Darton, Longman & Todd.

Chapter 7

Coping with change

As people face life-altering illness, they and their families will find themselves having to cope with considerable changes in their lives. Patients' sense of belonging is disturbed because they can no longer assume their roles and habits at work, in the home, or in the wider community. Somebody else is emptying the bin, organising the meals, and doing many of the other things they used to do, such as driving the car. Paradoxically, letting go of old patterns of doing and belonging in favour of new ways of being together can bring relief as well as times of frustration.

Denial and overprotection

The patient's and carer's perception of the illness changes, sometimes very suddenly. Some women who have had a mastectomy, for instance, cannot look at their scars and would not dream of taking their clothes off in front of anybody. Some partners cannot bear to look at them. Some women, after a while, may think about reconstruction, what that means and whether it would make a difference. Others still come to accept how their body looks and how they feel about it, with or without an implant. People's perceptions and awareness vary, as well as what they can cope with. Hence, in times of stress, both patients and carers can display a range of defences, the extremes of which are denial and overprotection. These can take many forms and occur in many different settings.

Most patients know that people do not always recover from cancer or serious heart disease. Thus the further forward they get from the diagnosis, disease, and treatment, the more confident they feel that they will recover. A delay of recurrence reassures them. It can confirm what they set their mind on believing; that the disease is no more than a hiccup and that they are absolutely fine. Some people deal with the illness in this way. For others an attitude of denial buys them time to get used to the idea and settle themselves to cope with the threat. Thresholds of denial vary greatly. A therapist comments: 'There are people who think about recurrence and the people who don't want to talk about it. One of my patients, Jim, had the treatment, had the surgery, had the radiotherapy, and his pain threshold must have been phenomenal because he didn't do illness; he didn't do pain. He didn't want to talk about it'.

The following story of Connie shows how denial and overprotection on the part of friends, family, and staff can be painful for patients, who may feel there is an invisible wall around them that they cannot reach out through.

Connie was a very young woman in her twenties. She was diagnosed with something in her lung when she was pregnant. She had the baby and died when this child was about four. She got to the point where she decided 'enough is enough', that she was not having any more chemotherapy and she was going to spend whatever time left she had at home, which she did.

Connie came into the department one day and wanted to see the doctors. She came to say goodbye, but they wouldn't—probably couldn't—see her. I sat with her. She was upset that nobody would talk to her about dying. All her friends and family were coming to visit, and she wanted to scream at them. Every time she tried to bring it up, but not one would say 'I have come to see you because you are going to die'.

She was beside herself with the near deception of the people that were coming. She wondered 'What do you talk about to somebody who has a limited life expectancy?' She had made her choices and had it all sorted. She knew where she was; she planned her funeral, she had made other preparations, but she was frustrated with people because they didn't know what to do when they came to visit her. They seemed unable to engage with what was real, which of course is hard for people when they care deeply about someone.

Empathy, vigilance, and time are needed to decode the signal and significance of denial and decide on the best way forward for all involved. A patient, known to one of us, has lived in the same village all her life and yet, now she has cancer, her lifelong friends do not visit her; some even cross the road when she approaches. She feels desperate and lonely due to their behaviour. Such attitudes are not uncommon among people who fear death and feel uncomfortable with those who are facing it. They do not know what to say.

When friends and relatives avoid talking about death and dying, they may well be trying to protect themselves from reflecting on an occurrence they cannot control. Working through the circumstances of a friend's chronic or terminal illness can be unsettling because it raises questions and anxieties about their own mortality, which they may come to deal with only in their own time and space. This may not always match the patient's.

We have found through our work that it can be helpful to drop a hint such as 'what do you fear the most?' It offers patients the opportunity to talk about their fears of death and dying. Families are often shocked at first, then surprised at what can emerge, and are often helped by being given permission to talk about the 'elephant in the room'. However, this does not always happen.

It can be disheartening at times for the care team to have to take proper account of the thoughts and fears of the family or the nearest and dearest. Alice, working with Nicholas, recalls such a situation.

When I went to see Nicholas he admitted he was terrified of dying. I reflected that back, helping him to see that this was quite a normal thing to happen, and inviting him to talk about it. I wondered whether he was terrified of the process of dying, or whether he was worried about being dead. Neither. He was terrified of dying because his grandson, who was about six months then, would grow up without knowing him. Nicholas was fully aware of what was happening to him. His wife was in complete denial and she wouldn't talk about the illness, sticking to 'No, of course you are going to get better' and this sort of thing.

I spent time with Nicholas exploring about his grandson. We looked at the photographs of them together. Although his grandson wouldn't remember him, at least there would be proof there that he had known his granddad. I suggested that there were things that Nicholas could do that would help his grandson remember him. I said, 'Have you thought perhaps with your wife of making a scrapbook, or a photograph album with a bit about your life, so that when your grandson grows up he will know some of your memories?'

By this point Nicholas was lying in his hospice bed thinking through his life, not able to write it down, but his wife could have done that and I said, 'Maybe you might like to write a letter to your grandson?' As we explored different possibilities, he became animated. When his wife came in I asked 'Would you like me to tell your wife what we have been talking about?' He did and I told her, but she wasn't having any of it. Now what could we do? He was going to go home and I guess they never did any of that.

For Nicholas, not being able to teach his grandson to play football and the idea of his first grandchild and grandson not remembering him was a source of great suffering. Yet his wife's denial of the severity of the illness, which was as much as she could cope with at that time, did not allow taking care of Nicholas' need. Had he been in the hospice longer, something could perhaps have been done to help both of them.

Sometimes denial or overprotection may come unwillingly from the wider social network. Alice, working with Andrea, tried to point this out to the local vicar.

Andrea had been a very active member of her church. She ran the Sunday School, had started the Old People's Lunch Club, and had been doing many other things. When she became ill in her late sixties, everybody said, 'There, there dear! You don't need to worry about anything, we will do that.' From being extraordinarily busy, everything was taken away from her. Andrea was aware that there were some things that she could not do, but some things she could.

That was an occasion when, as chaplain, I needed to ring her vicar and have a quiet word with him to clarify the situation, during which I suggested that Andrea could not stand and cook lunch, but she might be able to lay the table, or sit and fold the napkins, so that she could still be part of it.

Family and wider network relationships can foster or impede a patient's well-being. This can be due to a lack of information and awareness or because of problems they are struggling with themselves around the illness. We noted in the introduction of this book the reluctance of many to talk about death. Kaya Burgess in an article in *The Times* newspaper referred to research findings supporting that view. She quoted Eve Richardson, chief executive of the charity Dying Matters, who warns that unless we are more open in talking about death and dying, we will fail to get the desired and necessary care and support at the end of our lives. (Burgess, 2011)

Reticence in talking about death can further create major difficulties, for instance in failing to make a will. If this happens, and the person dies intestate, the legal requirements may require actions that would not have been the wishes of the deceased and family relating to inheritance. Another common consequence in failing to make necessary decisions at a time of death is confusion about the sort and conduct of the funeral. Our experience confirms that this failure to talk openly and make decisions about the realities of the situation is common and leads to misunderstandings and disappointments at a time when sensitivities and emotions are particularly aroused.

Interdependence and mutual impact

Illness can be the trigger for patients to inspire and encourage others. Chris ministered to Sophie, a young patient, as a chaplain. She felt safe in the hospital and her calm was a source and a resource for all at her bedside.

Sophie was a young girl of fourteen. Her mother was in hospital with her most of the time. She had a strong belief that there was a life that she was going forward to and she wasn't really concerned so much about the lack of time she had left in this life. She was looking forward to whatever heaven might be. We were amazed how she was coping and it was good just to be there and let her talk about how she felt.

Sophie had all the reassurance both from family and from the practical things and attention she needed from the hospital, where everything possible was being done for her. She felt safe and cared for. She wasn't alone. I sensed that her mother was more distressed and it must have been very difficult for her to put on a brave face when she was going to lose her daughter.

When I called in to see her, Sophie would give me a nice smile and be so welcoming it was reassuring for me. We were at ease with each other; we weren't anxious, we were not worried. She must have done the same for her family. In fact Sophie was profoundly calm about all the issues involved. She was sharing equanimity around and remained the still calm centre for all at her bedside.

Sophie's story suggests interplay of feelings and mood around the bedside. When the patient is quiet and calm it may be easier for family and staff to be with them until the end, although it does not take away the anxieties and the pain, which family and friends may wish to talk about. We have seen with Rebecca, on the other hand, how a patient struggling to accept the ordeal can put great strain on family and carers. In her determination to be at her son's wedding and maintaining her teacher and mother role, she denied her family the opportunity to prepare for her death. (see Chapters 2, 4, and 6)

Dealing with the sense of loss of usual and familiar ways and attitudes is never straightforward. It can lead to a necessity to cope with new circumstances and responsibilities for patient and family.

We are reminded of Albert, a patient suffering from a brain tumour who developed uncharacteristic behaviour at bed time and was at high fall risk. His wife, keen to avoid him getting hurt, felt driven to pre-empt any of Albert's needs and to spy on him. Albert was aware of his wife's anxiety, which heightened his own and increased his frustration. Sometimes they would get so worked up that they both ended up exhausted by the experience and deeply saddened by these uncharacteristic ways.

Coping with such changing circumstances can be immensely stressful for all involved and we see in these examples how the attitudes of patient and carer can be interdependent. Our attitudes tend to be mutually reinforcing, for better or for worse, and it can be very hard to break the cycle because of the complex emotions and realities involved.

That the attitude of one person can impact on the dynamics of a whole group is evident from the following story from a person-centred therapist facilitating an encounter group. The facilitator recalled:

A frail young participant named Amber announced within the first half hour of the group that she had AIDS (Acquired Immune Deficiency Syndrome) and that she was probably going to be pretty ill and could even die during the week.

'What did the group members feel about it?' The way she put her cards on the table had all the group members absolutely riveted and it was unanimously felt and recognised that such input was appropriate; this was who she was and that was how she was.

Amber's contribution to the group experience was profound. At times she became extremely frail and there were two or three sessions where she couldn't come and had to spend time lying on her bed. But her ability to make friends with her death and the strength that she got from the others, which increased what was already her great courage, was one of the most striking experiences the people in the group had ever had. It did not stop people from encountering. There were some difficult and painful things going on, but the overall context was one of almost blissful holding.

If anybody had asked me in advance 'What is it going to be like to have a young woman in the group dying of AIDS?' I would have been apprehensive. I might even have wondered whether to let this happen at all. But what did happen was that everybody faced not only her mortality, but their own. They were in an encounter group, committed to authenticity and, in the context of their corporate humanity, instead of fear there was peace.

Amber knew that she was taking a great risk of being rejected. But what happened was an almost immediate acceptance and validation of her state of being, which was in fact a state of dying. What she did by 'living her dying' in the presence of other people was an enormous act of faith in humanity, and all participants in that group felt validated. They responded by what the therapist called a 'blissful holding' of themselves and each other.

An encounter group is an unstructured group in which the participants seek to increase their sensitivity and emotional expressiveness by freely verbalising and responding to emotions. The assumption in encounter groups is that the individual will grow in a positive way by breaking out of social restrictions and by interacting with others honestly and openly.

In families too, attitudes and relationship patterns can change as a result of the experience of illness. Martha was a lady in her early sixties recovering from breast cancer. She had been caring for her husband—a heart patient—for the last ten years, and all of a sudden the tables had turned. Rachel, a counsellor, gave the following story:

Martha came to counselling because she could not understand why having done so well getting over the initial challenges of her illness, she was left with very difficult feelings. A lot of frustration and stress and anxiety had cut into her life, and a lot of anger seemed to be displaced on people who did not really deserve it. She was shouting at her husband and other people she loved most dearly.

Over the sessions she discovered the sort of person she was. She had always been someone caring for everybody else, like her elderly parents, who had died just prior to her cancer, and another elderly couple she visited every week. Martha was a pillar of the small village community and was also very active around the church. In addition, one of her daughters was at times rather insensitive in dumping the grandchildren on her, which left her looking after a toddler and a baby even though she didn't feel up to it.

Gradually Martha began to recognise her need and responded to it by being able to say for instance 'No, I don't feel I want to do that, I cannot do this at the moment.' She also recognised that she didn't allow other people to care for her. She didn't even let the family take on a caring role so they had given up on her.

As a result of the counselling this shifted dramatically. Martha was now crying with the family, and the girls rang her up every evening to ask how she was. She had been quite resentful and angry about her husband's lack of support and all of a sudden he was now bringing her breakfast in bed and finished off some room decoration. The woman who had just come out of surgery and chemotherapy and who had been decorating the spare bedroom was now being helped by her husband finishing the job.

Martha's awareness instigated a change of attitude, which in turn shifted her family relationships. This helped all in the family to participate in Martha's illness, and later in her dying, in a more harmonious and reciprocal way.

Facing a new future

The demands on people who have recovered from major illness in facing the future are often underestimated. Such changes can encompass physical and situational elements but also important psychological ones. Having expected to die and then to realise that one is not dying creates a fundamental new future. One could almost say a new birth. This can apply to the patient and/or to the family and they do not necessarily react in the same way. Such was the case for Nicole, with whom Jennifer worked as a therapist.

Nicole had a lot of issues to contend with in her life: she had been faced with a close bereavement, her son had been diagnosed with a severe mental health problem, her husband was having trouble at work and she was doing a very demanding job as well. A year of chemo and eight months off work had given Nicole time to think. She had started up a little business and was wondering how to keep this going when she would go back to work; she needed her full-time job because of the family's financial situation.

Nicole looked well, and as it so often happens, her family and friends thought she was back to normal. She felt they expected her to be normal, and she wanted to be seen as such. Even during treatment or following surgery, Nicole tried to look well. She didn't want any kind of special treatment, pity, or sympathy, although it was nice to have the support. But when Nicole had managed it through her treatment, once she stopped looking ill, she felt that what she had been through was all forgotten. The children became quite demanding again, and her husband was still on thin ice about his job and his future. She was a bit sad, or angry, that there was this expectation of her to start doing everything as before.

Sometimes Nicole wanted to say, 'But I may not be here next year!' She had been dealing with life and death and had had painful chemotherapy and other people's problems seemed quite trivial in comparison. Nicole struggled with this transition. She was not a patient any longer but she was still feeling anxious and worried about becoming a patient again.

Nicole, like other former patients, had to face the challenge of having a future and what to do with it. Would she go back to where she was before this happened? But the experience of illness had changed her. She had become more sensitive; perhaps more self-centred about her feelings for others, or sometimes she was just so tired she could not make it to the end of the day. Yet she was back to expecting (and being expected) to care for others when she still needed care for herself. Trying to do everything she used to, she was absolutely exhausted and became angry and resentful when this was not picked up or accepted.

Needing to integrate two different worlds, former patients can feel very lonely. They may find it difficult to cope with their ambivalent feelings and even harder to express them and put them across. They oscillate between wanting to leave it all behind and enjoy living, and worrying that it may all come back. Similarly, family and friends would like to get on with life and forget it ever happened, sometimes as a way of fending off their fear of an uncertain future as their confidence, too, had been shattered.

Unfortunately the oscillations of expectation that patients, family, friends, and carers feel are often not on the same wavelength or beat. They may find it difficult to empathise with what the other is going through. 'Lets get on with life, you're well now, what is there to be afraid about, consider yourself lucky' or 'Don't be so over-protective, I want to get on with my life' are not unusual. In struggling to come to terms with personal fears and anxieties, there can be little space and energy left to attune to the other, and being out of phase with our nearest and dearest can be lonely, painful, and distressing.

It can take some time for patients to adjust to the world of illness and hospital dictating their lifestyle. Readjusting to life after illness is a challenge too. Even when there appears to be no change—for instance home is still the same house, the same children are there—they can be perceived as different due to a changed outlook. We know of a patient who was discharged from hospital to her own home. She was convinced that her bed had been changed because it felt different. However, it felt different because she had lost so much weight and her new bony frame changed her experience of it.

Having come through the ordeal of treatment successfully, some patients still carry residual grief and pain. The illness may have upset habits and functions in and around the family and that too can be painful and unsettling. Change rarely comes easily; it can even be met with significant resistance. Patients are faced with the challenge of reformulating the questions 'Where do I belong?' or 'Who do I belong to?' into 'Where can I be?' and 'Who am I?' A challenge it is, but one that we have seen can bring hope, peace, and fulfilment.

References

Burgess, K. 2011. Questions about death left unspoken. The Times, May 17th p. 13.

Chapter 8

Some personal consequences for the carer

The focus of care is, quite properly, on patients. All the primary resources are organised to respond to their needs. However, the whole network of support relies on the motivation and well-being of the carers, both lay and professional. In this chapter we consider some of the personal dangers for carers that can affect sufficiency and competence, and some of the consequential rewards.

Fatigue and self-neglect

Many times throughout this book we have drawn attention to the existence among many carers of the reality of exhaustion or weariness. This phenomenon can apply to both professional and family carers, but probably for different reasons. The professional can become overburdened by the sheer weight and variety of the caseload, which will include the growing number of older clients or patients needing regular support and whose dying does not leave them untouched. The increasing expectations, sometimes quite unrealistic, can also induce a sense of failure and hopelessness.

> *A district nurse who was off work because of depression shared her concerns that she could no longer face a list of patients who often waited longingly and impatiently for her visits as if she was a sort of angel of mercy. She realised that in practice, she could not meet their hopes and expectations, as she could do so little for these people in practical terms to relieve their suffering and especially their loneliness. Her depression revealed itself in a profound tiredness, fatigue, and 'lassitude', which captured the physical, psychological, and spiritual aspects of her situation. This would barely be reduced by a good night's sleep. Subsequently she reported that even that was denied.*

Such a sense of burden is perhaps all the more common among family carers, who live permanently and very close to the major or chronic illness of their loved one or friend. We have already described the range of practical tasks and responsibilities that major illness can impose on those who are required to be the frontline supporters, generally without training or preparation. Even so, what often makes it really tough for the family carer is their enormous emotional involvement with the patient and the whole family situation. The role can be so demanding that it can threaten the inner resources and capacities, not only of the carer, but of the whole family.

Fatigue is a symptom or sign of many things, including major illness, but it is commonly a sign of continuous and excessive work, which can reduce the ability to function normally or sufficiently. There may be physical indications such as aches and pains, muscle weakness, sleeplessness, and stomach disturbance. There can also be psychological signs such as depression, eating disorders, general weariness, boredom, and sharp mood swings. It can indicate emotional stress, which can be a common concomitant to the constant caring for a very sick or disabled family member. Such circumstances can induce fatigue and negative attitudes, which can damage relationships as well as the standard and style of care, sometimes even tragically to the point of including personal violence and abuse. The carer can feel trapped; the patient feels a victim of circumstance, tensions rise, and solutions seem very distant. Even hitherto strong relationships can be undermined and become fraught.

It is evident that emotional and psychological stress, which at times seem so understandable, can lead to ineffective team working between the carer, other family members and friends, and the visiting professionals. Love, loyalty, guilt, and the denial of realities can all be powerful constituents to a misplaced and excessive commitment, which can endanger the carer and in turn the very special thing the family carer is committed to supplying. As carers become fatigued, all sorts of other things can so easily go wrong, including the carer becoming ill themselves.

Fatigue is a subtle assailant and one often not recognised until it begins seriously to affect the standard of care or the carer's well-being. Despite a natural tendency for the professional carer to focus attention on the needs of 'their' patient, we feel that an important part of their role should also be to watch over the lay carer's well-being. It could be necessary for them to warn the lay carers of the dangers of excess and to try to put in place ways of protecting them, even from themselves. Similarly, friends and other family members have a responsibility to advise, care, and encourage breaks by offering to assist in covering the time when the carer is off duty or on holiday. We do not consider this to be a diversion from the care for the patient but an indirect function in preserving it.

In addition to fatigue and in spite of external help, many family carers of all ages experience a sense of loss of freedom, friendships, and outside contacts. A possible consequence of the carer's total focus on the patient can be self-neglect. The habit of eating regularly and sufficiently, ensuring proper sleep and exercise, and taking time off can fall by the wayside. One of our interviewees called her limited free time 'me-time'. She insisted it was necessary and she achieved it by retiring to her bedroom behind a closed door. If such self-care is not undertaken, then there will be a strong possibility that the carer will become exhausted; physically, mentally, and spiritually. The overwhelming routines can become destructive and lead to bitterness, sadness, resentment, and boredom. alongside a drop in the standard of help for the patient. Such was the case for Hannah:

> Hannah married Gerald late in life. Five years later, Gerald was diagnosed with motor neurone disease. Hannah was there for him in every way. Caring so intensely while Gerald's condition deteriorated meant that her world contracted steadily but surely: Gerald did not like leaving the home so they did not go out together any longer. She gave up meeting with friends to be with him and look after him. She became so exhausted and fatigued that she had to be signed off work with depression. This dragged her into despair. She loved her work, which was her 'escape' from an increasingly demanding husband and patient. She needed to feed him and as he would refuse to go to bed when the carers came in to help at 7 pm; she felt forced to do the job herself. This she increasingly resented. She felt blackmailed. Their relationship was strained by the caring and the expectations, and as a result the standard of care and mutual understanding dropped.

In such circumstances, it would not be surprising if the relationship with the patient deteriorated. Tempers could become frayed, attitudes to each other more rigid and fraught. Conversation could be inhibited, quite apart from the restrictions imposed by the illness or pain. Many within the patient–family carer relationship find it difficult sharing their true feelings with each other when conditions are good; but when they are not, such important questions as 'What can I or should I say?' 'Will I make things worse or not?' become profoundly problematical or even impossible to consider or discuss.

Self-neglect, despite the provision of regular supervision and staff support, is not uncommon among professional carers. Clinical depression, addictive behaviours, compassion fatigue, and burn-out are but some of the visible consequences of self-neglect. Yet, for the professional, as for the lay carer, the emotional cost of caring for the very ill can weigh heavily on marital, family, and other responsibilities.

For the family member, the sheer grind can also result in depression and a sharp drop in quality of care, whatever may be the feelings towards the patient. This in turn can induce feelings of guilt. Self-concern, far from being selfish, is vital for the well-being of both carer and patient.

Guilt

Guilt can be focussed on many aspects of caring. As we noted at the beginning of the chapter about demands on the family, people often become family carers suddenly, without any planning or training. They are pitched into a life change. A sense of guilt about the quality of care being offered is common among family members. They are probably doing their best, and most patients recognise this when they think about it objectively. There can also be strong guilt feelings when the carer recognises that they are falling short in their efforts, even if this is imagined. They are longing for relief from the routine. In many situations this longing is natural, but the sense of resentment at the situation still weighs heavily upon the carer. This is particularly so when there is a chance that the illness has been brought on by the patient's own behaviour, such as smoking or drinking heavily. Some form of blame is understandable, but carers may still feel guilt from nursing such feelings or even more actually confronting the patient with them. Forgiveness in such circumstances is enormously difficult, because people feel even more guilt at their lack of capacity to forgive. Nevertheless, forgiveness could be a huge assistance in creating a supportive and positive relationship if it can be offered and received.

A feeling of guilt is not always rational. It can be based on a sense of inadequacy or failure that cannot be supported by objective facts. It can be a sort of referred pain.

> One of us experienced a relationship between a couple that was scarred by the conviction of the woman that the demands of her illness had caused the demotion of her husband at work due to his concern for her and his caring of her. In fact, the reason for his demotion was his difficulty in coping with the demands of new technology. She based her conviction on her need as a paraplegic to be especially cosseted at weekends when her husband was tired and at home. Her husband responded willingly and he was adamant that this gift to his wife had no influence on his fate at work.

The supposed impact of her illness and her guilt about it was objectively out of place, because it related to her husband's work problems.

One of our informants talked about not knowing what was really happening or what he should really feel. He felt guilty because he was not as depressed as he felt perhaps he should be. He also considered that he had not given sufficient of himself to his ailing wife while at the same time holding down a very demanding job. 'I do not deny the future. I currently ignore it. That is my way of coping, insufficient indeed, and I should do better' he said.

Carers, like patients, can endure a cocktail of emotions, including anger, frustration, resentment, as well as the opportunity to show love, care, gratitude, and hope. This contrast and conflict of motive and feeling is itself a drag on the sense of vitality, the loss of which leaves many carers feeling guilty and trapped.

Loss

In caring for patients with life-altering or terminal illness, a sense of loss comes in many guises. It emerges as a powerful psychological response to dramatic change, from diagnosis all the way to death itself. Death is of course universal and we considered the social responses to it in the Introduction. However, losses of one sort or another occur all the way through life. Some might be considered 'big losses', others are little ones. A 'big loss' could be thought of in terms of a loss of a spouse or job, of mobility or eyesight or mental capacity. A 'little loss' may be something that hinders previous ability, such as no longer being able to play golf or walk without a stick. Yet whether one experiences a loss as big or small is a very personal thing and a big loss for one can be much smaller for someone else.

> *A widow who cared for her bed-ridden husband suffering advanced dementia was asked why she seemed not to mourn in the 'usual' way after he died. She replied that she had been mourning over eight years as each of her husband's losses of capacity occurred. His passing was accepted in her terms as a 'divine mercy'. 'There will be no more (losses).'*

Losses are associated with change or endings. And as they become more frequent or significant, their effect on those concerned can become increasingly threatening and generate further demands on carers.

A subtle but often overlooked aspect of loss comes with the realisation that the person in one's life who is loved for himself or herself is no longer the person originally met. One of our informants, who said that her husband 'is no longer the person I married' and that 'the children have lost the father they thought they had', felt that she was serving a life sentence. Two other informants spoke of the greatly increased challenge that such circumstances produced. The loss of mental faculties such as memory and awareness can seem to the carer to be inexorable and a heavy addition to an already difficult task. An informant who cared for a cancer patient who had also developed Alzheimer's described it in common parlance as a 'double whammy'. Thankfulness on the part of the patient is no longer expressed; conversations about their past relationship or the conduct and meaning of their lives is no longer possible. For the carer, there is the problem of not being able to assess truly what the patient wants or needs.

Silence or incomprehensibility dominate. A relationship is lost at a time when it is perhaps most needed. In spite of this, the length people will go to care for a loved one or family member, a willingness driven by love, faithfulness, determination, or a sense of duty is often remarkable. Such carers need all the help they can get and we would suggest that the outside professional help is all the more relevant in such situations.

Rewards

The picture of personal consequences so far given appears to be one of unmitigated challenge and disruption. In some senses this is accurate to describe such a life change for patients and carers, but it is not the whole picture. The challenges are real and powerful, but the experience of so many is that all is not lost. We can still look back, around us, and forward to see that there is life to be lived in spite of a number of high hurdles to be overcome. In spite of everything, serious illness, while naturally feared and disliked, is seen in many circumstances to be the conduit of growth and new understanding.

Philip Gould, one of the architects of New Labour in the 1990s died of oesophageal cancer in 2011. When he found himself in what he called the 'death zone', he became upbeat. He told Andrew Marr, who wrote about it in *The Times* of 8 November 2011, that it was the most extraordinary period of his life as well as the most significant. He went on to assert that if one could accept death, fear of it would be overcome. Not everyone would describe that time in those terms, but what is often recognised is the added value it brings to time itself, to relationships, to the beauty of nature, and to the past experiences of one's life.

There are often similar feelings among family and professional carers. Amidst the grief and stress, there can be thanksgiving for the time given to grow different quality relationships and to see the qualities in that very special other person. It can be the time to respond to them with love and care, commitment and a very particular form of closeness, sometimes not unlike that of a mother with her baby.

Such a time can also be one of growth spiritually, and for some like Philip Gould again, a fresh and developing sense of the presence and power of God can be discovered. The gifts each of us have been given may become almost fluorescent; they stand out in a way hitherto not seen. The relationship can warm and deepen.

One of our informants, while recognising the things she found stressful and limiting, was grateful for the time she could care for her husband although it had never been a marriage of deep love. Somehow, his needs unlocked the gifts she could offer, and she, and perhaps he also, felt liberated as a result.

In this aspect, the different and yet coherent coordination with professional carers can become especially valuable. They offer their friendship, skills, experience and objectivity, which can fit well with the family carer's gift of devotion, love, and sensitivity, which only a person who deeply knows the patient can present. The combination can bring a powerful blend of care for the patient and indeed all the carers, from whatever position they come.

Part 3

The professional carers and their roles

Chapter 9

Challenges for the professional carer

We have considered some of the major issues that come to families and friends as they react to the onset of a major illness for one of their loved ones. As we have seen, these challenges can stretch the family resources, and the need for help to cope becomes ever greater as the illness progresses. In response to these needs, there is a small army of professional carers working in and from hospitals and hospices and in the community to bring personal support and professional skills to the aid of families. There are nurses, therapists, doctors, counsellors, and trained volunteers available, and all make their contribution. Like the family carers, they too have specific challenges as well as those common to all who seek to support the very ill. The range of issues is significant and as varied as one would expect, with almost endless possibilities because they cover relationships, both one to one and multidisciplinary, and reflect personal backgrounds. These present to us such questions as: 'What characteristics facilitate the development of an effective and satisfying caring relationship?' 'What are the implications of patient-centred care for the professional?' 'How can we differentiate between roles?' 'How can we manage boundaries?' Some of the more common are now considered.

Patient-centred care

While care should be primarily focussed on the patient, we want to emphasise 'patient-centred' care, by which we mean treating people as unique and whole individuals, not as objects to be cured. This approach is sometimes referred to as 'holistic' care, meaning that all aspects of the person (physical, social, emotional, and spiritual) are brought into the equation. Thus patient-centred care is not limited to the patient. It takes into its orbit the whole family; it may even address the wider social network.

An essential quality in patient-centred care is empathy: the capacity to enter into the patient's world without losing oneself in it. The following story shows how Alice's empathy and alertness helped in solving a problem for all the staff dealing with Peggy, a 72-year-old dementia patient who had been in hospital for over a year.

*Peggy and her husband had moved to France when he retired. They were hav-
ing a lovely time and then, as so often happens when people retire, he dropped
dead. It was absolutely devastating for Peggy. She appeared to be mentally ill
and was sectioned under the Mental Health Act.*

*Peggy had spent much time coming to the chapel, sometimes putting flowers
there on her husband's anniversary. One particular day a gentleman had come
in to see her and he was very alarmed because he understood that she'd been
absconding. He asked her 'Why do you do it? Why do you go to the cemetery?'
'To look for my sister's grave,' she said.*

*The nurses didn't know about this. They hadn't thought to ask why she went.
So I explored it. It turned out that Peggy had four older brothers and sisters.
Her mother was then pregnant with another child after her and they were out
one day and a horse pulling a delivery cart reared up near her mother, frightened her, and sent her into premature labour. The baby only lived a few days
and mother was distraught. The baby was buried at the cemetery and Peggy
was going there to look for the grave. She said her mother was really distressed
and used to take her up to the grave and used to cry a lot and she remembered
some flowers going on.*

*I found out where the grave was, had the grass cut back and then one morn-
ing one of the staff nurses and I escorted Peggy up there and we had a short
ceremony which did a lot of good. Prior to going, Peggy was in a right state,
which is how she gets. Afterwards, she was extremely elated and we were able
to say to her 'Now look, these are your landmarks. There is this particular tomb
with a horse on top of it, you go down the path there...' With the map she
would be able to go herself when she was allowed to. It hasn't cured her, but
I think with her there is so much bereavement work to do that it's going to take
a long time, but I believe that this was one of the steps.*

Peggy had a very severe bereavement problem, with identity connotations that
impacted on her overall condition. Alice's empathy and patient-centred reflection guided her attitude. She guessed how important it might be for Peggy to
go to her sister's grave and have a ceremony to acknowledge that her sister had
lived and been buried there. Peggy would now be able to go to the grave on her
own without having to abscond. The whole process gave her landmarks about
who she was and her personal and family history.

The nature of empathy is very different from sympathy. One is so close
to the client that it is as if one were in their shoes, but one is not taken
over by them. Empathy is often more difficult for family and lay carers who
may be overwhelmed by the pain and distress of their loved one. Sometimes
an empathetic connection can be manifested in unexpected ways, such as

an emotional response. The therapist can cry and genuinely share the pain they feel. It is a therapeutic skill and a challenge, rooted in the therapist's self-knowledge and self-awareness, to be present both to the client and to herself and discern whether an emotion or bodily sensation they experience is theirs or whether it reflects the client's feelings; and if it is the latter, to use this insight in the therapeutic encounter. This clarity about what is one's own response and what is another's is very important for true empathy.

In our understanding, caring is best understood in the context of relationships. These encompass both professional and lay people, who are all subject to different disciplines and organisational codes of good practice as well as the traditions and culture of the family and its circle. If we want to offer patient-centred care we need to be aware of the whole person. This can be enhanced in a multidisciplinary team. For optimal functioning, the professional team faces the challenge of achieving adequate and appropriate communication between its members and with the patient and family. They need to share necessary information with the appropriate people to enhance and support holistic care, whilst respecting the confidentiality of what has been entrusted to them.

From the stories of our informants, we have found that challenges frequently emerge as relationships with the carers are forged and conversations and therapy develop within the framework of trust. They are not theoretical or hypothetical, but real and often powerful. Some are straightforward, others complex: some confront the carer as a professional, others as a person. Some will be relevant to specific carers, others will not, but all will be relevant to the people who have lived or are living the experience. On the face of it therefore, the complexities underlying these relationships bring demands and challenges to all concerned. Narrative accounts can serve as a point of learning and inspiration for many others travelling their own journey.

Finding a common language

When working from a patient-centred perspective, one of the first requirements is to be able to communicate with the patient. Empathy is a necessary condition but finding a common language can still be a challenge, as the story of Rachel's work with a teacher in his late forties makes clear. Cyril had made good recovery from a sarcoma but the statistics for his type of cancer were not good, and he knew it. Back at work and doing everything he could to keep fit, he was not holding together emotionally. His consultant suggested that he seek counselling. Rachel reported:

The first meeting with Cyril was hard work. His clever, academic way frightened me. He told me of the medical history and the pressure of having to go back to work, but I couldn't help him acknowledge his feelings associated with that. In the school holidays we had a much easier time. However when he went back to school, I found the next session was more difficult. I felt at the end of my tether with this man and had prepared a list of the names of counsellors and agencies who might be of greater assistance to him.

And then we had an amazing session. There was this rush of connection and warmth between us. He opened up about his family relationships and the difficulty for his wife of having to live with the uncertainty of the diagnosis. Right at the end he said: 'I want to tell you something, I've never told anybody this'— and proceeded about his regrets for something that happened 25 years ago.

Dropping the idea that she had to sort things out for Cyril and match his intellect, having even considered sending him on somewhere else, freed Rachel up to be more relaxed, and enabled Cyril to connect and share. Rachel reflects:

This man was going to very deep places on his own and I was just beginning to get glimpses of that. He didn't want to wallow in 'what if's' and 'getting ill or getting better'. There was a part of him that knew that it was there, but he was doing it in a different way. He talked about applying for another job, wanting the quality of his life to be different, wanting time for other parts of himself.

He wasn't making obvious statements about death and dying, but everything about him was addressing it and I could respect that, following and staying very close to how he wanted to address it. At the start I didn't have a language with him, but we were finding one.

Rachel felt that she was failing because Cyril did not address his feelings. She was intimidated by his intellectual language until she realised in that pivotal session that he did a lot of the 'feeling' work in his own way and looked to Rachel to be a witness and a sounding board.

In finding a common language both therapist and client progress. Therapy is a joint exercise in which a meaning is sculpted, which for both is new. It is the product of the ability to work together when the client is both heard and understood (Fessler, 1983 p. 44).

Creating and holding a safe space

When our professional informants were approached about the exercise of their care, they were asked questions about what they aimed for with their clients or patients and how this coloured their encounters. Some goals they mentioned were about the type of relationship and the space they tried to offer.

Alice, a chaplain, tries to meet a patient with an open agenda. Her aim is to go where the patient wants or perhaps needs to go. She finds useful the metaphor of 'entering a pothole', similar to one used by Edith Campbell, a chaplain who worked with people with HIV and AIDS. She used to describe her relationship with her clients as companions on a journey into unknown territory. She did not know where they were going to take her. They had the map, set the pace, and, if they wished, walked into the depths of a pothole. Edith metaphorically held on to the safety rope while staying on the surface. The client could explore the depths relatively unhindered. Journeys into such depths were found to be a vivid way of psychologically experiencing our deepest selves; but knowing that another holds the safety rope brings freedom, hope, and direction. Alice finds this analogy helpful:

> *Spiritual care is a bit like the person who maintains the safety of a potholer, holding on to the harness while the potholer does whatever one does in the dark at the bottom of the pothole, and then when he is ready, pulls him out again. This requires mutual cooperation and trust.*
>
> *I guess my aim is based on that because the teacher and the nurse in me might want to tell them what to look at down there, but actually I need to let them look at what they need to look at in that moment and to feel free to talk about it.*
>
> *Spiritual care is very much the patient setting their own agenda. It's allowing them to explore the bit that they are looking at right now. Because I'm not there and they are down there, the viewpoint is going to be different. With hospice patients who are ill those encounters may be quite short. The end result is for somebody to find peace and tranquillity so that they can relax and hand over.*

The professional carer needs to create a space in which the patient can find their own answers. We can be tempted to suggest our answers, but it is more helpful for the patient to find their own, and they may often surprise us. Allowing a patient to talk things through and hear what they are saying helps, especially as not many people really listen and patients may not have experienced being listened to in depth before. Encouraging the patient and their family to face the sometimes difficult reality, with its challenges and opportunities, can be hard work; so is staying with the pain, especially when it is very raw. Being alongside someone in the bleak black hole demands courage and perseverance on the part of the carer. The same need for creating and holding a space applies to lay carers, especially family members.

Jane, a doctor and psychotherapist, tries to let patients know that what they say and feel is acceptable. It can be a time to air anger, sadness, humiliation, and also a time to teach the patient about their illness and how to handle it.

This provision of space may mean an empathetic silence—the therapist stays with the patient in their thinking. Creating such a space takes time and commitment. Jane comments:

> As a doctor I check how they are sleeping, what their understanding of their illness is, try to find out what they are afraid of, debunking things that they fear that are not going to happen and promising that we will be there for them for things that are likely to happen.
>
> As a psychotherapist I try to build up patients' self-esteem, telling them that being ill or dependent doesn't make one a lesser person. I talk to people about their relationships, because that is usually the most precious thing for people, and their relationship with God if that is an issue for them. I suppose I try to bring people through to an acceptance of what is happening.

For many families there is unhappiness and sadness, and to lighten that burden and offer a little bit of joy may help them find some peace.

As we have already observed, patients and carers may respond to the circumstances of critical illness with a sense of weakness and uncertainty. Promoting healing therefore involves a significant task towards inspiring feelings of courage, hope, determination, and a sense of control. To this end Billy, a social worker, sees his role as facilitating, giving permission, giving information, and bringing in and mobilising resources. More than anything else he aims at harnessing families' inner strengths, giving them the tools and the means to decide what they want to do, and whether and how they want to do it. It is his role to strengthen families to make the decisions that will affect them. He considers himself an enabler and commented on his work empowering a family in his case load (the story of the Lambeth family is recalled in Chapter 11, 'Talking about illness in the family') to develop more satisfying relationships despite the illness:

> I suppose the work is about helping the family members to be role-appropriate. Thus we happened to empower Joseph, the ill father, to say and to identify his needs, and actually enabled him to feel that he could be a dad—not just focus on his own needs.

Rachel, an individual therapist, empowers patients by trying to get to their resourceful side and develop it. She helps patients to create a map of what might be helpful for them and to tap into it. What goes into the map to discover an appropriate route can be as varied as information, emotional resources, physical exercise, and other things that can help them manage uncertainty, belonging, faith, and spirituality.

For Siobhan, the important thing working with people with chronic and life-threatening illness is helping them to manage their complex situations better. They need to reconsider their personal and working lives, and this comes at a cost to their feelings and sense of self. A particular resource in this is seeing other ways of harnessing those feelings, especially anger.

> Siobhan herself had complicated feelings about anger around illness which took her years to work through. She recalls how she started off by feeling sorry for herself. Then she asked: 'Why has this happened? What has happened to me? What have I done? I haven't done anything to deserve this.' Subsequently her attitude shifted in the light of increasing understanding. She had been angry, but did not realise it, and she recognised that she had to learn that process to be able to discover her true feelings.

Having learned to decode her anger she looks for similar signs in the clients she works with. To this end, artwork is one of the skills she uses to bring feelings to the fore and explore them. She reflects:

> I used to consider anything like art therapy very airy-fairy. I had to let go of my fear about things like painting. Sometimes people dealt with their anger and fear, as in diabetes, by going out and buying sticky buns or donuts, and then their diabetes was all over the place.
>
> When people become aware of their anger they can use it positively to help them eat and do the right things. Question is, 'What can you do instead?' but it starts with accepting myself, why I have to eat this cream bun, even though I know it doesn't do me any good. It's a very long process of bereavement, anger and resentment, that ebb and flow. Acceptance is never totally achieved. It's a process of coming and going.

In nursing, as in counselling, Siobhan feels that it is important to sustain people when they are feeling desperate, probably lonely, and in pain, by staying with what is and just being with them in that moment. Staying with these feelings may allow fresh thoughts to arise. Patience is the key; the issue is the journey, not when and how it will end. What is the patient going through in that time? It is in the journey as well as the arrival that learning and movement are experienced.

Flexibility in approach and response

In *Dying to Talk* Heyse-Moore (2007 p. 11) underlines how the complex nature of life-altering illness demands flexibility. Such flexibility helps to ensure 'security' and 'well-being' for patients and families and is a necessary requirement for effective multidisciplinary teamwork. As part of the multidisciplinary team, psychotherapists and spiritual carers are in a position to give people time when medical staff are often so busy that they cannot spend long with each patient.

Jane, a former consultant and now a psychotherapist, made the poignant remark:

> *I've been used all my life [as a doctor] to working with people for five or ten minutes at a time and I never thought that I'd be able to tolerate spending an hour with someone.*

While there is an objective issue about the time that people can make available, the ability and preparedness to give people of our time is also a challenge both for the professional and lay carer. It can vary according to personalities, to people's sense of their responsibilities and to how they are feeling at the time.

While giving their time is part of what therapists and spiritual carers are there for, the amount of time they can or should give in the palliative care setting is not straightforward. Counselling sessions traditionally last for 50 minutes to an hour, but people with terminal illness do not have the strength for long conversations. Most psychological work with people in a hospice is done in ten- or even five-minute doses, and instead of a weekly appointment, daily input is often needed at critical times. Sessions tend to come to a natural conclusion. Sometimes, at the other extreme, an encounter or a family meeting—shortly after diagnosis for instance—can go on for two or more hours.

Patients do not need psycho-spiritual care the whole time and they may not necessarily need it when a visit is made by the chaplain or therapist. They may on one day but not on another. This lack of contractually assigned time may put a strain on the therapist who might, for instance, refrain from going on a ward round shortly before a multidisciplinary team meeting to avoid getting caught in personal conversations that cannot be governed by such boundaries. Patients' and families' sense of timing may not coincide with that of the organisation or with the therapist's other commitments.

> *A chaplain was about to go on her way when Lester, a patient returning from an outing, unexpectedly invited her over. He jumped straight in at the deep end with his question 'What is death?'*

Lester's attitude illustrates the notion of 'subjective experience of time'. It could be that he had been wrestling with this question for a while, and seeing the chaplain made him express the question that had been on his mind. What felt untimely to the chaplain, who did not want to bother Lester who (she thought) might want to rest and recover from the outing, felt to him like the right moment to tackle this important question.

Further to considering the time issue, the setting in which counselling takes place carries its own challenges on carer flexibility. When we are talking to a patient in a bay with four beds, confidentiality may be compromised, even though drawn curtains may provide a feeling of privacy. Often other members of staff or a family member are present and it is not uncommon for one of them to change the subject or answer on behalf of the patient.

> *The encounter with Lester changed when his wife Sheila appeared. A conversation that started at the deep end talking about death, changed direction when Sheila joined in the dialogue, determined to talk about Lester himself and his weaknesses. Suddenly the chaplain had to shift focus to accommodate the needs of both spouses and how they related to each other. Sheila's outburst of anger and resentment was unexpected, and her denial of Lester's condition added to his pain. This happened in the bay and was witnessed by three other patients and their families.*

The holding presence of the chaplain provided safety. One may wonder what happened at the meeting she missed as a result of being alert to Lester's needs!

While the physical setting can constrain the counselling relationship, the psycho-spiritual space one can offer in a patient-centred encounter should not be downplayed. Louis, a doctor involved in medical training, told of some striking experiences of students to whom he had introduced the idea of giving the patient psychological and spiritual space. He explained:

> *One of the most effective things was having students going off, either in pairs or individually, to the wards where they had been working for a couple of weeks and have them ask a patient two sorts of questions. One of them was: 'What keeps you going when things are difficult?' 'What are your sources of strength, courage, hope, etc.?' 'How do you deal with adversity?' 'Where do you go for help with that?' The second question was 'Do you think of yourself in anyway as religious or spiritual?' They were then asked to clarify what they meant by that.*
>
> *The students usually came back pleased with what had happened. One said 'I came away thinking for the first time ever that I had actually helped somebody'. Two other students had interviewed an elderly woman and said she kept talking about love and they had the feeling that people's eyes lit up while they talked about what sustained them.*
>
> *There is this kind of healing energy that is awakened by giving permission, as it were. And almost all of the patients said: 'Nobody has ever asked me about this before', and yet one might say, 'Well my church has been so important to me, it's really nice'.*

The medical students were amazed at the depth and extension of connection they experienced with some of the patients around whose beds they had stood more than once without a hint of anything beyond their pathology, symptoms, and complaints. Similarly, the patients felt honoured and enlivened at being given that space to be who they were. They no longer felt like children who were bossed about according to medical orders; who they really were as a person had become significant for this 'doctor' who came to ask them about their life's experience. The first set of questions offered a way into exploring patients' inner resources and strengths and the practical and emotional external support available to them. The second question opened a door to their spiritual dimension.

Patient-centredness demands focused listening as well as appropriate attention, where one softly and openly offers something to another; the more so because the hospital experience tends to make patients feel that all initiative and control is taken out of their hands. Respect for the other's private space means not trespassing beyond their boundary, but also going the distance to meet them at that boundary rather than standing back where we imagine it to be.

Coping with a backlog of grief

Therapists' experiences have brought to the fore the emotional investment of professional carers in their relationship with patients. As a former Macmillan nurse, Rachel told the story of her first experiences of supervision, which makes explicit the build-up of grief that carers in this area of work may have to carry.

> I was a Macmillan nurse before it became the norm that specialist nurses had supervision. All at once supervision was on offer and it opened for all of us a huge well of things we had not dealt with about the job; most of the time we spent sobbing. There was a huge backlog of grief and loss to work through. Some people couldn't cope with this; they stopped going to supervision.
>
> For me being able to talk about the loss was a revelation which played a part in my moving on to becoming a counsellor. It wasn't unusual to have six deaths a month out of my caseload and either you have a clearance system in place or you have to tuck it away. I'm still drawing on all that loss. There is still residual stuff there for me. It doesn't get hugely in the way now, but it deepens my empathy.

The professional's grief reflects that of the patient and their carer, but is compounded by repetition. Dealing emotionally with six deaths a month asks a great deal of people, and there is not always the right support in place to help them with this or what support there is may be overwhelming or difficult to access. Some of the Macmillan nurses Rachel referred to were snowed under when they addressed their backlog of grief, while the very nature of their work required them to be fit for more work, facing more death and dying an hour later.

There is an issue here about what society provides for the people from whom it expects so much. On 27 February 2009, at a time when Catherine was working around this issue, she heard the then Lance Corporal Johnsson Beharry, the youngest person to be awarded the Victoria Cross, expressing a concern on the part of some serving soldiers about the lack of aftercare and support for men and women who have left the armed services. In particular he was concerned about the lack of psychological support for the trauma they had experienced. It is curious that a little short of a century after the First World War revealed the devastation of post-traumatic stress disorder, we still have not grasped the fact that these incredibly traumatic events have often disabling long-term effects.

In Western European countries people have become more comfortable acknowledging trauma and its lasting effects than they were in 1918. Nonetheless, little attention is paid to resolving them. In a range of occupations, such as the medical profession, the fire brigade, the police, and the army, the capacity to suspend immediate emotional response and take action is required. The Macmillan nurse deals with people who are dying every day and continually has to work through or—as is more often the case, keep setting aside—their own feelings and questions about death and dying.

How is it possible to remain caring in such circumstances when feelings must be set aside? Rabinovitch points to this paradox, questioning whether money is wisely spent on teaching communication skills to doctors (Rabinovitch, 2007 p. 27). We could legitimately ask whether it is possible and right to train such professionals as doctors, paramedics, or police officers in the arts of empathy when we also expect them to operate with appropriate detachment in a crisis. Detachment could be considered to be the opposite of empathy—and to expect both in critical situations could create a stress over priorities to the detriment of both the 'helper' and the 'victim'.

We do not seem to have found a way to come to terms with the fact that in order for some of our society's services to run smoothly, we require people to pretend that things do not affect them so that they can do what they have to do. The situation is helped by supervision and talking groups that are now offered in most palliative care services, but some staff need more or different ways to help cope with stressful work. It is not surprising that, on average, people work in palliative care for only about 12 years, and they come to it later in their lives. It appears that still more attention needs to be given to support to carers, given the reasonable assumption that in the long term it is not good for people to have to keep putting their feelings aside in order to be able to do their work.

Taking care of themselves

It is difficult to overstate the importance of self-care. As we reflected on such dangers for lay and family carers, we need to realise that professionals are not immune from the consequences of stress, overwork, or a sense of lack of support. Carers walk a tightrope, balancing the need for closeness and the worry of not being able to cope. They need information, help, support, and advice to equip them for their role. They also need to remain fit and able to confirm and encourage what brings life when helping patients and families to work through phases of anxiety. What helps carers take care of themselves? Eve said: 'Often what helps the patient helps me'.

Working in this field, the energy does not all flow in one direction. There can be a mutually healing and helpful process between patient and therapist. Rachel shared the satisfaction she gets from her work with cancer patients:

> I get so much out of the work because I meet people at a time when spirit is apparent in them. You see it both in the person with the illness and in the people around him. You see resources demonstrated which often they themselves do not recognise or know they had. To me that is 'spiritual', and the incredible thing about the work is that you see that part of people live.
>
> They may be people who don't talk about God nor believe in religion but even then, the end of their life is the end of the line. What's healing at that time is the connection from spirit to spirit; a connection with somebody—it doesn't have to be me, it can be the family, a carer, a chaplain, a friend. Facilitating patients' capacity to connect helps them cope with the pain and the situation, clearing the things that are getting in the way, getting through anxieties, stresses and depression; clearing a jungle to get through to the person for whom experiencing that connectedness is healing.

For Rachel it is clear that there is a reward from her work that nourishes her. She feels that she has to take care in order to ensure that the mutuality is about the journeying together and not about meeting her personal needs. The privilege of seeing the deep inner resources of people unveiled and experiencing such rich encounter demands a proper ending. Rachel said:

> It felt important to have an ending with Olivia. I had my own sort of ending, some private time, but I think it would have been helpful for me to go through the more formal processes of the funeral. I was on my way to work when I saw her coffin and the family assembling as I drove past. It was unsettling because I wasn't going to be part of it. Ending can be different for every person. It's about finding what expresses your relationship with that person.

Indeed, each ending will be different and one can understand that doctors, therapists, and nurses do not attend all the funerals of the patients in their care. Chloe suggested:

There is an ambiguity about ending. When we don't do it, it's not always that we are ducking out of a response. It can be that we don't need to. Similarly some family members are full of regret—'I wish I'd said goodbye' or 'I wish I'd told him I loved him'—whilst others are okay.

Sometimes it may seem to be right to attend a funeral, while in another instance a card, a letter, a candle, or some private prayer or recollection is more appropriate.

An often invaluable experience of support for professional carers happens through encounter and connectedness with colleagues and professional supervisors. Billy said:

Without that regular and solid supervision, I'm not sure I would have done the quality of work that I was able to do with the Lambeth family. Supervision allowed me to stop and stand back, to reflect and take stock and then plan the kind of options that were open to me as a professional to engage.

Talking and sharing about the work is important. Several research participants said that even our interview with them had the quality of supervision because it allowed them to talk about their experiences and process their feelings. However, supervision is not enough. Professionals need to find their own individual and institutional ways of taking care of their emotional needs to prevent compassion fatigue and burnout.

References

Fessler, R. 1983. Phenomenology and the 'talking cure': research on psychotherapy. In: Giorgi, A., Barton, A. and Maes, C. (eds.) *Duquesne Studies in Phenomenological Psychology*, Vol. 4. Pittsburg: Duquesne University Press, p. 44.

Heyse-Moore, L. 2007. Dying to talk. Therapy Today **18**, 11.

Rabinovitch, D. 2007. *Take Off Your Party Dress. When Life's Too Busy for Breast Cancer*, London: Pocket Books.

Chapter 10

The power and limitations of words

Struggling to put our experience into words and honouring the voice of interviewees and patients, we have often resorted to metaphor to put across deeply personal and rationally indescribable experiences. Words are among our most precious gifts to point to the wonder and mystery of creation, beauty, desire, compassion, and our common experience of suffering. Sometimes words fail, yet words can find striking, universal images. Thus poetry, as Heaney (2002) suggests, is pitched between things as they are and as they could or should be. It encompasses the disappointments of reality, and remains, as hope, an indispensable part of being human. Images, metaphors, and stories have a better hope of capturing some aspects of the mystery that lies in and around us.

Buber (1937) writes about the potential of a story to convey a new truth, bring about change, and liberate those who hear it. There is a long tradition of the human need to convey and discern truth through images and stories, as in Wagner's *Ring of the Nibelung*, C.S. Lewis's *Narnia*, J.K. Rowling's *Harry Potter* or Tolkien's *The Lord of the Rings*. Metaphor, symbols, and stories are tools for touching life at its deepest level. Yet their understanding may still differ between people and require interpretation of what each understands it to mean, an invitation to dialogue.

Beyond words...metaphor and symbol

In an effort to arrive at a truth about their experiences of life-transforming processes, patients and carers often turn to symbol and metaphor as tools of storytelling. The word 'symbol' is derived from the Greek σύμβολον (*sýmbolon*, meaning 'to connect', literally 'to throw together'). Many examples exist. Perhaps a powerful one is a flame, which can symbolise warmth but also the danger of burning. A candle can provide light, but it can also be a sign of sacrifice and extinction as it burns down. In another way, a piece of cloth can be a flag, a symbol of national pride, unity, or determination. A symbol cannot only be very specific but can also encourage thought and recognition of associations and ideas that convey a meaning well beyond the basic fact of the symbol itself.

When we speak about one thing in terms that are evocative of another we use metaphor, in Greek μεταφορα (*metaphora*—transferring meaning from one word to another). A good metaphor therefore can convey complex thoughts and feelings with impressive economy. It 'invites interpretations from many angles' and 'there is never an exact literal equivalent' (Stanworth, 2004 p. 19). However its meaning is often easily recognisable in the context.

A metaphor offers a way of expressing thoughts and feelings that can perhaps be said in no other way. This may be why it is a regular feature in work with the chronic and terminally ill. Trying to find an image of common experience can help to bridge the comprehension gap between carer and patient. Jane, a former consultant, shared how she tried to demystify a patient about her illness and symptoms:

> *A young woman, Naomi, came to see me who had a cancer of the cervix. She had her uterus removed, but the tumour had come back and she had a frozen pelvis, which meant that the tumour had grown into her pelvis and her organs were stuck together, which caused a lot of pain. Naomi kept asking: 'Why can't they operate?' I explained: 'Do you know about polyfilla? If you mix that in a cup and you leave it, it'll go completely solid. Cancer in the pelvis is like polyfilla in a cup, you can't take it out without breaking the cup'.*

Using the metaphor of polyfilla in a cup, Jane explained the illness in language the patient could understand.

In person-to-person communication, metaphor creates safety and allows people to take a conversation to quite a deep level and at the same time ignore the subject or treat it lightly. People are not put into an uncomfortable position or forced into a corner.

> *Rachel, a therapist, was wondering why Beth, a woman with cancer of the ovary, would spend a whole session talking of a disaster story about repairs to her house: she was getting the wrong washbasin, the pipes did not fit, and nothing ever went right. Beth talked about the bathroom for an hour; towards the end of the session she would cry and the metaphor would become real for her. What they were really talking about week after week was the chaos of this woman's life. It took Rachel a while to recognise that Beth's bathroom worries were a metaphor for all that was going wrong in her cancer-ridden body.*

Many of our professional informants felt that their best work happened when they invited people to respond at the level they felt they were at. Saying something like 'I guess you've had a big change in your whole lifestyle' allows a person to ignore it or to say 'Yes, my life has been turned upside down', or 'I don't even have the energy to do the ironing or wash the children's uniforms'.

In his dealings with patients, Billy, a family therapist, recognises what he calls 'double talk', a way to describe a process where the counsellor and client may be talking about something at many different levels. There is a switching back and forth between factual conversation about medicines or information about help or resources and something quite deep. Billy comments:

> Doing homecare I find myself commenting about the garden and talking about the pain of not being able to keep it as nice as she or he used to, even just watching in silence, making an affirmative comment about how nice the garden looks.
>
> With bereaved people the garden is often a focus of conversation: 'He isn't there now to do it' or 'That's his favourite rose coming up'. In terms of prognosis and approaching death, sometimes there is this element of time about looking forward: 'I'm going to miss the beauty of these plants and my familiar garden'.
>
> I throw out seeds of thought and see if anything comes back and what does. Some people say 'Oh, I don't want to be upset' and give a clear, direct signal that they don't want to go there today.

Billy uses metaphor to open a channel of communication. A metaphor can be a trigger or a subject in itself. People can stick to the garden or they can take the hint at what next year's blossoming represents and their anxiety about that. Billy's use of metaphor is a mark of responsive respect, i.e. a willingness to go along where the other wants to go. Such willingness to talk about ordinary things, but which can convey deep meanings, is a tool open to lay carers as well as professionals, for they could be in a position of actually sharing, for instance, the garden with the patient.

The metaphorical language of rituals

Many simple gestures or words, such as lighting a candle on a festive table or sending a birthday or a Christmas card, support daily life and emphasise the meaning of daily events. On the other hand, important events and transitions such as birth, adolescence, graduation, marriage, and death are marked by major culturally-defined and embedded rituals. They have a personal and a collective meaning.

The metaphoric language of ritual consists of symbolic words, but even more importantly of gestures and symbolic actions that mark the change being celebrated, as for instance, the exchange of rings in a wedding. Rituals are a means of communication and can offer a mixture of both clear understanding and wider interpretation or experiencing. When a judge enters a courtroom, for instance, all stand up. This is a ritual, but also a symbol as we stand up for what the judge represents, not for him as an individual.

Sign, symbol, and ritual are culturally defined. A metaphor, grounded in physical experience, can transcend cultural boundaries, understanding, and construction in a similar way to mime. It can be a very powerful means of communication between people who do not share a common language. We refer elsewhere (Chapter 2, 'Relationship and communication' and Chapter 12, 'Chaplaincy and spiritual care') to the significance of holding the hand of very ill or dying patients. A connectedness is literally made, and can symbolise so much to a person who may be feeling profoundly alone.

Rituals not only add splendour to an event; the ritual itself also supports the changing reality. After the ritual has taken place, the individual is no longer the same (Leijssen, 2009).

> *A person known to us experienced this recently: returning home after four years in Norwich, she felt drawn to clearing her house of all the things that she had kept for so long because she could not decide what to do with them or where they belonged. Clearing the clutter felt like a ritual expression, a symbol of the transition marking the change she had experienced over those four years; owning and inhabiting her environment accordingly supported the change and brought security and a sense of freedom to move on.*

Leijssen (2007) points out that big and small rituals are about connectedness, about being part of a community, about creating an atmosphere of safety in difficult transitions. They remind us that ups and downs are a shared experience among people. They are about raising hope that there is something larger to fall back on, and about enabling transformation. Rituals bring the healing that lies hidden in the origin of traditional habits into everybody's reach.

A ritual can be helpful to support change and transition, as for instance when a client brought a picture of her deceased husband to a therapy session to express what she regretted not having had the opportunity to say, thus helping her to let him go. One of the gifts of chaplaincy is that it can ritualise a meaningful event and so help patients and their families to mark a significant occasion or become clear about something. Alice, a hospice chaplain, tells the following story:

> *There was obviously something troubling Carmen. She had a lovely husband who used to come trotting in each day, and twin daughters who were in their forties. One day she asked to talk with me and said, 'Actually my twins were triplets, but they don't know that'. I invited her to say more. The twins were born, and all was fine. A few days later Carmen started to bleed heavily and passed what was thought to be a miscarriage and she said 'And that was the*

little boy'. As happened in those days, it was just taken away and burned. Forty years later, Carmen felt that she was mother to that foetus and that it hadn't had a funeral and she needed to come to terms with that before she died.

There wasn't a vast amount of time, considering how poorly Carmen was, and after talking about it, I offered to have a little service where this little one was acknowledged and she gave him a name. Her husband obviously was aware of this little son, but the twins weren't and Carmen wanted to tell them. This was a bit of a shock. I did an order of service, Carmen and her husband were able to read a little prayer, 'And we name him…' and until the day she died she held that piece of paper with his name in her hand. It got very messy, but it was precious.

Although apparently moving on with one's life, unresolved issues can linger and may come back to the fore at some significant time. Knowing she was dying, Carmen needed to acknowledge her son's existence and after the ceremony, the little paper with the name they had chosen was a precious reminder that she kept till the end. Similarly, Alfred, who would not make it to his daughter's wedding, was able to give her away during a tailor-made ritual and ceremony.

Alfred was very poorly. His daughter was getting married and he wasn't going to be able to go and give her away and he really regretted that. We managed in the hospital to devise a little service whereby he could give her away to her intended husband. Alfred actually went up the aisle in the chapel, he in the wheelchair with his daughter to give her away.

Alfred, as a father of a daughter, believed it was his duty and privilege to give his daughter away and despite the circumstances Alice provided an opportunity for him to do so before he died.

Beyond communication, encounter

We have already considered the challenges of communication, which can go far beyond language. Doctor Jane commented on how haphazard communication can be, 'There is no formula for working with the dying' she said; 'you never know whether what you are going to say is going to be right and perfect, or very wrong'. Her encounter with Moira exemplifies how the effect of a conversation can be surprising.

There was an elderly lady, Moira, who was blind and she had cancer. She was due to have her cataracts operated on privately and because we thought she had only another week or two weeks to live the nurses said to me 'You can't let that woman go for surgery at this stage—it isn't worth it. You have to tell her.' I went in and we had the following conversation:

> Dr Jane: *I'm not sure you really need this operation (I hoped she would say 'Yes, I realise that')*
> Moira: *Why?*
> Dr Jane: *Well ear hasn't heard, eye hasn't seen, nor has the heart of man conceived what God has revealed to those who love him. I think in a short while you will see very well.*
> Moira: *But Doctor, I've been so wicked.*
> Dr Jane: *Oh, what have you done? (This was a woman aged 75)*
> Moira: *When I was young I was very beautiful and I managed to seduce the husbands of my two best friends.*
> Dr Jane: *Oh, right. Would you like to go to confession?*
> Moira: *Yes.*

It was Monday and there was no Catholic priest about so I got the local Anglican priest who came and heard her confession and afterwards she said 'I feel at peace with everyone'.

How unexpectedly and quickly a conversation can change direction or depth! Jane came with the difficult agenda of delivering bad news. Inspired and using a Bible reference at her second attempt, her message came across and suddenly Moira jumped to another level of conversation. This is a good example of how spiritual care is not only in the hands of chaplains or spiritual carers; it is the responsibility of the whole team. Jane heard Moira's question and her offer to call in a priest was welcomed by the patient.

For many, personal encounter is the great opportunity to move on, as Louis experienced as a young psychiatrist. He was very keen to get through to Jeremy, a patient whom the staff found difficult to engage with.

In this particular ward several people were not responding to treatment, particularly Jeremy, who used to moan, cry, and weep. He couldn't speak in coherent language. I wanted to spend time with him; I thought there had to be a way of getting through to him, something I could do. I went back several times to see him. I talked to him but didn't know whether he could understand me.

On this one particular day, the last time I saw him, I was really frustrated at not being able to communicate and help him in some other way. I was lost in thought trying to think of what to say or do next and not willing to give up when he came up behind me, put his hand on my shoulder and said 'Let's go and have a cup of tea!' And then he just wandered off!

> *To my knowledge, he had never engaged with anybody in that way before.*
> *I thought: 'He's the one who is taking care of me now.' I felt humbled that he*
> *should suss out that I wanted to help him but I couldn't. He was saying in effect*
> *not to worry, somehow it was all right. I recognised that profound communica-*
> *tion can go on between people of which none of us are aware sometimes.*

Jeremy's attitude is reminiscent of Ella (see Chapter 4, 'The part of life one
has not lived'), who appeared to wake up after days in a coma to thank her
therapist. Both tell us never to underestimate a patient's awareness and capacity for connection and communication. This is why nurses are taught to talk to
unconscious patients they are nursing.

A psychotherapist who spent 20 minutes in silence with a client experienced
its potency. Julia had been working at a deep level, closely in touch with her
grief. Her pain was raw. At its heart was the statement 'I have given all my
strength away; I have none left to help myself'. The therapist's interventions
were sparse. One she remembers making, shortly before she realised something
special was going on, was along the lines of 'I am touched by how much love
you have to give and how generously you have given it'. Julia did not reply. She
was staring intently at a point in the distance. The therapist recalls:

> *Julia seemed to be listening to or communicating with something or someone.*
> *It occurred to me that she might faint or be unwell, but my overall feeling was*
> *one of deep intensity and presence, which I felt called to respect, privileged to*
> *witness such a potent moment. I could let it be and be with it, fully present to*
> *the client and to what was happening in the silence. When she finally spoke 20*
> *minutes had elapsed, but it had not seemed long, so intense was the experience.*
> *A bit shaken and shivery, Julia said:*
>
> > *'I feel weird…Where did this come from?…How did that hap-*
> > *pen?…I was looking at that button on the coat and suddenly…I don't*
> > *know where it came from…my strength was given back to me…and*
> > *I feel so different now…it feels like a big burden has been lifted from*
> > *my shoulders…I feel so good now…I could run…What has hap-*
> > *pened?…Where did it come from?…'*
>
> *The client looked at me for answers, for understanding, but I did not know*
> *what had happened and was careful not to take anything away from her*
> *experience by bringing in my own frame of reference. To meet her unease*
> *I said: 'Looking at you, I have an image of a spring from which a boulder*
> *has been cleared and the water flows more freely'. Faithful to my sense*
> *of mystery, the metaphor offered a handle without limiting the client's*
> *experience.*

That something can happen in the silence is very clear from the account Julia wrote after the therapy of the day she saw 'a vision in the button':

> *This Wednesday started as usual talking about the last few hours of my part-*
> *ner's life, the things I had done to make his last few hours comfortable. Across*
> *the other side of the room was a coat lying on the chair with three or four large*
> *buttons; one of these caught my eye as if it wanted to tell me something. After*
> *about 45 minutes I was very upset but drawn to this particular button when*
> *suddenly it sent something to me; strength? And also something that took away*
> *the sadness which had built up. I wanted to laugh, shout, and skip away.*
>
> *My partner had always said that as soon as he had enough strength at half-*
> *way house where he would wait for me, he would send me my strength back by*
> *being with me in spirit. I think that is what he did by way of that button. From*
> *this moment on I have felt different, able to be me, do things for myself, and not*
> *be in that washing machine churning about. I still have that room deep inside*
> *me when I feel sad, and I am sure it will always be there for me to take myself*
> *when I need to have time alone with my memories of someone so close. People*
> *talk about miracles. I am sure this was mine.*

Brian Thorne, a person-centred therapist and writer, probably described some-thing of this therapist's thinking and attitude during that 20-minute silence when he wrote about 'magic moments' when client and therapist experience a 'waiting without expectation but also without despair' (Thorne, 1993 p. 75). Encounter engages people through deep and sensitive channels, way beyond speech or physical demonstration. Even silence conveys messages. Part of a good training in counselling should include the capacity to listen intently and with understanding to what is not said as well as what is.

References

Buber, M. 1937. *I and Thou*, New York: Charles Scribener's Sons.

Heaney, S. 2002. *Finders Keepers: Atlas of Civilisation*. London: Faber.

Leijssen, M. 2007. *Tijd Voor de Ziel*. Tielt: Lannoo.

Leijssen, M. 2009. Psychotherapy as search and care for the soul. Person-Centered & Experiential Psychotherapies, **8**, 18–32.

Stanworth, R. 2004. *Recognizing Spiritual Needs in People who are Dying*. Oxford: Oxford University Press.

Thorne, B. 1993. Spirituality and the counsellor. In: **Dryden, W.** (ed.), *Questions and Answers in Counselling in Action*. London: Sage Publications, p. 75.

Chapter 11

Talking with patients

Communication involves information, facts, and data but also feelings and perceptions. The hugely complex nature of communication accounts for flaws and failures. These are mostly not due to ill will or even negligence, but cannot be taken lightly either. Informing and communicating with patients and their families is an area in which huge improvements have been made. Michael Mayne reflects:

> A senior consultant, who taught my surgeon…warns me that I may feel low in the coming weeks, not to put on a brave face but to let my emotions emerge, not to be afraid of tears. Unlikely that a senior consultant of even ten years ago would have expressed such views. An encouraging shift…Here is a man trained in a different medical tradition, prepared to adapt to new insights about how his profession most effectively communicates with patients and seeks not just to convey a sense of confidence in its medical skills, but to address them as persons at every level, body, mind and spirit (Mayne, 2006 p. 160).

Conveying a sense of confidence in one's skills is important to reassure the patient. But Mayne strikingly reminds us that it is not enough. Patients feel the need to be addressed as people. Hence, when and how to give appropriate information is a permanent challenge, and there is room for improvement, as in the example of the nurse who was going on holiday and said to the patient 'By the time I come back you will feel really horrible'.

Breaking bad news

Although knowing the truth of one's situation can be important, timing as well as tact and sensitivity make all the difference to whether and how a message is received and understood. Sometimes, hearing news, even bad news, can bring relief so long as it is conveyed with gentleness and compassion.

> *A recent example of how not to break bad news was given to us when a consultant told a very sick person: 'It is bad news. You have got cancer of the brain and a few weeks to live'. He then left the room.*

In this encounter, the patient was not 'met' as a fellow human being but as an object not even worthy of encouragement or pity. What a contrast to the senior consultant who warns the patient that he may feel low in the coming weeks and encourages him not to put on a brave face.

Information should be conveyed with sensitivity and, if possible, by someone who knows the patient and their strengths and weaknesses. In all cases, the task requires skill, experience and an in-built instinct about the patient's capacity to cope. When these essentials are missing, there can be misunderstandings and serious negative repercussions. It is vital that carers recognise what patients are going through and how sensitive they are to fears and assumptions that do not have any factual base or are exaggerated.

Sharing information

A further example indicates the danger of a failure even to share information at all, as well as not doing so with sensitivity.

> *A terminally ill patient was removed from a three-bedded room in a specialist cancer ward to a side room without explanation. When we met her, she was in a distressed state because she was assuming that her condition had worsened and that she was nearing death. In fact, when asked, the senior nurse told us that the patient had been moved because the space occupied by her bed needed clearing in order that the floor covering could be renewed.*

Nobody had thought of telling the patient the reasons and so she suffered considerable and unnecessary anxiety.

In the doctor–patient relationship, problems of communication can occur when the patient, out of fear or ignorance or because they do not want to be a bother, fails to share what they are feeling or their symptoms. Patients are often surprised when they are told that the medical staff need their help by not holding back any information about their symptoms or pain. Potentially bad news can cause the patient to turn in on themselves, hoping that the problem will go away. The doctor's approach of kindness, patience, and skill in asking the right questions can free up the patient to entrust his information to the practitioner. Carers of all sorts can, with the correct attitude, get alongside the sufferer and allow for a natural, open relationship to develop to everybody's advantage.

In all these communications and relationships, the watchwords are sensitivity, tact, courage, gentleness, honesty, patience, and to do the loving thing. This will allow for the feelings of all involved to be heard and respected. What is ultimately vital is that the sense of vulnerability of patients is reduced, and that they do not feel alone as they struggle with their disease, but loved, respected, and understood.

Helping people to be heard

What helps to get it right when talking to patients is empathy and respect for and understanding of each other's perspectives. Sometimes a simple thing can be overlooked. This was Rachel's feeling about Annette, whom she saw in therapy.

> *Annette had worked all through her chemotherapy and seemed to be getting the message from the medical profession that she shouldn't be doing that. But it worked for her: it was a distraction, she said. She had worked for the company for twenty years and the people were fantastic, very understanding. I encouraged her, and though it was such a simple thing I did, it was a huge relief for Annette, and I was so sad that it hadn't happened before.*

Annette was getting over breast cancer and reconstructive surgery, but was still in a period of uncertainty with fears and thoughts around the illness. Continuing to work had been normalising for her, but she kept receiving worrying messages from the medical staff who—perhaps out of their own professional anxiety or personal perspective—felt that she had better stop working.

Patients need to be honoured for what they try to do and experience. Work made this woman feel alive and healthy, and that was precious. Rachel, Annette's therapist, said 'It often doesn't take much', meaning that Annette only needed someone to recognise her endeavour and her judgement to feel relieved. The professional opinion of her continuing to work needed to be made clear too as an important bit of information and a reality check, but in the end it was Annette's life and her choice. The lack of recognition from the people she looked up to as 'experts' left her feeling guilty and lost.

Just as Annette looked for a witness to her efforts and the decisions she was making, Benedict felt that Arthur (see Chapter 3, 'Inner turmoil') wanted to bounce ideas and discuss strategy while he was trying to build more effective relationships with his wife and son.

> *What seemed helpful to Arthur was to have a place to report in about what he was now managing to do. He enjoyed having a man-to-man relationship and the carapace seemed to be gradually melting away. Trying to create different kinds of relationships with his family members, he was mirroring that with me and probably in many ways being aided by it. Once or twice, at his own suggestion, he brought in his wife. He wanted her to meet me as the arbiter and witness of the progress and effort he was making.*

In this part of the work Arthur somehow considered his therapist as a life-coach. He was trying out new things and wanted a witness, someone to report to and to discuss strategy with. Providing such support is not the role of the therapist as such, but it can be an advantage to talk things through with someone who is understanding but not directly involved.

Talking about illness in the family

Billy was involved with the Lambeth family as part of a home care team. While the nurse was concentrating on Joseph's symptoms, she had realised that his wife Annie needed support, and asked Billy to intervene. Annie was caring for a very sick husband and was trying to keep three children going—an 11-year-old boy suffering from asthma, a 10-year-old girl who had threatened to leave home, and a 7-year-old son. There was little extended family support and a lot of family conflict seemed to hinge on the illness.

> When I phoned Annie she welcomed help but insisted that the children should not be told that dad had cancer. 'The only thing I have managed to do is not to tell the children and I never cry in front of them' she said. I suggested that we have a family meeting and we agreed a time for me to come with the nurse who had made the initial visit.
>
> When we knocked on the door, Annie opened and said 'Joseph isn't well, he's in bed.' She looked exhausted. Thinking on my feet, I felt that the family needed to confront some of the issues together and said 'Is there any chance that you could go up and ask Joseph if he could come and join us, even for a little while?' She went to the sitting room with the nurse and then Joseph appeared and they came in and all sat down.
>
> I started off by: 'It's good to meet everyone. We know from the work we do that when one person is ill in the family, it does affect everybody and we were just wondering what it was like for all of you'. Then there was this huge silence and absolutely nothing was said for a long while. Eventually the youngest blurted out 'I hear Dad getting sick at night and I get upset.'
>
> The outcome of that first family meeting was that we were talking to each one about how the illness affected them and what their thoughts were. The parents agreed that I met with the children separately for a few occasions, and the nurse would focus on the symptom control with Dad. The nurse and I would meet with the parents from time to time.

Annie was worried about the children being upset and Billy felt it was critical that the team had the parents' support for the work he was doing with the children. He was trying to palliate the ignorance and fear in this household and he wanted to address the feelings and enhance communication in the family. He met the children four times, making use of an activity such as drawing, sculpting, or completing sentences in order to draw out the discussion. They explored beliefs and myths about the illness such as 'Cancer isn't catching',

'There's nothing you said or did or didn't do that gave Dad cancer', or 'You can't get ill because you're bad'. Through the sessions with the children, more and more hopes and fears emerged:

The youngest drew a sketch of each person of the family with huge tears dripping down Mum's cheeks. Even though it wasn't talked about openly, the children were aware. I tried to convey that it was acceptable to feel that the whole world revolved around Dad's illness and that they were never taken out any more; that they could still laugh and go on an outing and at other times be really scared and crying.

Billy helped the children to mention the unmentionable; he put into words some of the things that were going on. Expressing what they were feeling and thinking and being given permission to be the way they were was healing.

By Billy's third session with the Lambeth children there had been a lot of progress: the rows and the threats from the ten-year-old girl had diminished, the asthma attacks were under control, cancer was on the agenda, and they were talking about Dad dying. Given that the children were extremely bright and insightful, Billy felt they were in a way parenting their mother. Annie could barely cope. She was hyper-anxious and always busy. Billy wanted to help her be a mother again and allow the children just to be children.

By the third or fourth session I said to the children 'You know, I wonder how it's going to be when Dad dies. How do you think Mum will be?' The two youngest ones said 'Oh Mum will commit suicide'. This really shocked me. I wasn't expecting that response. I didn't even know they knew the word suicide. I was almost tongue-tied.

It transpired that there was a lot of mystery around grandfather's death, Mum's dad. It sounded as though he had died in the Holocaust, and one of the family secrets was that Granddad had committed suicide. That was how the children had picked up this word.

The children's worry about who was going to look after them threw Billy off balance and he wondered how to take this further. He had this contract with the children that what they did together was confidential. But trying to keep the parents engaged and to work through them, he also had this agreement that when he met the parents he would talk generally about the kind of work he was doing with the children. His supervisor suggested he called another family meeting and enabled the parents to say to the children what arrangements they had made.

We had a very emotive, sad meeting acknowledging that Dad was going to die and facing the fact that the children were worrying about Mummy dying as well. The parents handled it very well and said what arrangements were made if the children needed caring for.

Out of that meeting, we were talking about how to best use the time they had, together as a family. One of Dad's big regrets was that having been ill ever since the seven-year-old was small; they had missed out on getting to know each other. He would love to have time to tell him stories. We gathered suggestions as to what the family might do to help Dad and his youngest son to get to know each other. Mum and the two other children agreed that they would make a space for Dad and Christopher to spend time together.

On my last meeting with Dad he said 'It has been the best morning of my life, I had such a lovely cuddle with Christopher and it was just right'.

Families do what they feel they need to do in terms of sorries, thank yous and goodbyes in their own particular way, but in terms of helping parents be parents, Billy and the home care team's intervention enabled Joseph to retain or reclaim control when everything was out of control. Empowered to identify his needs and to feel that he could be a dad, Joseph could have, in bed, this wonderful morning with Christopher with the backing of his family.

Billy carried on working with the Lambeth family for a few months following Joseph's death. It was not a happy family. The rows went on. The girl had been the apple of her dad's eye, and she was absolutely hateful to her mother after his death. Billy helped them look at their relationships with each other and asked what, if they could have a magic wand, they would change.

One key thing was the ten-year-old girl. Something was troubling her, her anger was not standing on its own, it was rooted in something. We did a bit of writing with the heading 'If only...I wish we did or did not do something.' She wrote 'I wish I had a time machine and could go back in time' and 'I wish I had made Dad go to the doctor, I might have stopped his cancer.' We talked about her feeling responsible for Dad, who was having back pains and wouldn't go to the doctor, and she wished she had forced him. She ended her piece of writing by saying 'But even then, I don't know if it would have stopped the cancer', bringing in a bit of reality.

It often happens that children feel responsible for their parent's illness or dying. Billy allowed these difficult questions and guilt feelings to surface and helped them to understand their meaning. In the first contact Annie had expressed her belief that a good mother should hide the father's illness and her own distress from the children. Sometimes beliefs can be on the edge of awareness or unconscious and it can take time and creativity on the part of the therapist to help them to surface, as Billy did with the Lambeth children's beliefs about illness and cancer.

Chloe, a nurse and family therapist in training, at times felt completely helpless when working with Laura and Pete. Retrospectively she realised that some of the things she did were helpful. Laura's brain tumour diagnosis came about when she was thirty-one weeks pregnant and had a fit. The doctors knew they would need to start radiotherapy immediately and they had to have her baby delivered. The baby was small and went into special care, when Laura was just coming round to the whole idea of having a life-threatening illness. The staff nurse had realised that Laura's husband Pete was struggling and called Chloe in.

> *Pete was very diffident about my being involved because by the time Laura came home from hospital they were having a number of professionals coming in and out of the house. I met them for the first time when Laura was getting over the effects of radiotherapy. She was on high dose steroids, had put on a lot of weight and physically was looking very different from how she had been some time before. Pete was trying to manage a sickly and frail baby as well as a toddler. He was doing a lot of physical work and taking a great deal of responsibility for looking after the whole family.*
>
> *We had several sessions talking about the impact of illness on their life. A bone of contention between them was that Laura was relying on her mother to do quite a lot of supportive work and Pete was feeling excluded from this. There were issues about how they were functioning as a couple, as they tried to adjust to the illness. I was getting stuck with these two very different points of view, which they were giving me but not sharing together. Laura would tell me her story and Pete would tell me his version of what life was like and they were not engaging at all.*
>
> *I asked them to draw a circle that represented their life and to put different circles into it representing all the things that were important. That might be the people, it might be things that fed their soul, it might be anything; and to put in illness, and also what was happening from a physical point of view. I also invited them to make sure that they put themselves in there. What was fascinating was that the biggest circle in both their drawings was around the disease, but Laura described it as, 'Getting better,' and Pete as, 'Illness.' It became very clear when they looked at each other's drawing that they had no common language for talking about what was going on. Laura had put in her circles her husband, Pete, her two children, and her mum, but her mum was bigger than her husband. Pete had put his wife and his two girls in the drawing, but he refused to put himself in because he said, 'I don't exist'. The drawing was a very*

powerful way for them to be able to look and see what was similar or what was different and how we could try and help them to share more.

They had been describing about their life before as a very cohesive, loving, demonstrative couple and the illness had completely changed everything. They had been preparing for a second glorious child and instead they had illness and the extra child was almost an additional burden rather than a joy, although that was not ever made explicit. The tension between Laura and Pete, the sadness and the rift between them, was almost palpable. Laura had very little physical energy, but when she did have some it was expended on the children, especially the older child, and on her mother in phone calls. Pete didn't mind the lack of energy and the priorities that ensued, but he was feeling excluded. He believed that when you get married you are responsible for each other and you separate from your family of origin. Their different belief systems were causing friction and it was sad and difficult. Pete had been told information about Laura's long-term outlook, but she didn't want to hear it. She was talking very optimistically about getting better and he knew that whatever they did, the chances of her surviving more than two years were really small.

When Laura had a recurrence, she ended up in a medical consultation where she was given information without her requesting it. The doctors were so used to dealing with Pete who had been saying, 'Tell me how it is, I need the truth,' that they assumed that both partners were on the same wavelength. Following this we had some very painful sessions where Laura came much closer to Pete's worldview of what was happening. It was hard for me as a therapist to know whether that was a good thing for Laura. My concern was that exposing this together might create distress of a level that I couldn't contain; my fear was mirroring Laura's.

We see how different belief systems made it difficult if not impossible for Laura and Pete to understand each other and communicate openly. They needed help to see that although the illness was *the* huge thing in both of their lives, Pete looked at it as a disruptive 'illness', Laura as energy and time engulfed in 'getting better'. Another striking disparity in beliefs was Pete's focus of attention on mutual support, as in 'when you marry you leave your family to attach to your spouse', as opposed to Laura's looking to her mother for support.

Laura and Pete's story also brings to the fore how people perceive and accept things at differing pace. Earlier we considered the importance of timing. In talking to patients, this is crucial. If we want to be patient-centred we need to be aware of how the patient is experiencing time. If information is pushed at them, they may feel that their psychological space is being invaded and may not be receptive to it or may be frightened by it into a sense of helplessness. It takes fine-tuning from the carer to perceive the right time and the right way to give sensitive information.

Laura and Pete's story further highlights how therapist and carers share the patients' and families' concerns and difficulties in dealing with the truth about diagnosis and prognosis. There is no clear-cut answer. Twenty years ago doctors were trained and instructed not to tell patients. Now the trend is the opposite, yet, as we see with Laura and Pete, there are issues of best judgement about what the patient and family can bear and what will help them, as well as how to best communicate bad news.

Talking about getting better was Laura's way of coping and keeping the pain away. When she was eventually confronted with her prognosis both she and Pete had a difficult time. Still, it seems this was a pivotal occasion because it released Pete from the burden of keeping a secret. He was able to talk to Laura about how he wanted to share life with her; they could both look in the same direction. Their story echoes research findings that in dealing with cancer-induced changes, effective communication between spouses reduces conflict and role-strain and promotes cohesion and mutual support (Vess et al., 1985, 1988).

Chloe wondered whether knowing the prognosis was a good thing for Laura, as she was aware how painful and hard it was for her to face dying with two little children. One day Laura and Pete were really cross with each other:

> Pete complained, 'Laura's doing nothing with the baby, I have to do all the work. She'll do things with the older child, but she won't do anything with the baby. I'm tired and fed up with all of this.'
>
> I made an intuitive guess, and asked Laura whether it was quite scary to do things with her baby daughter. It was indeed. It was not the practical things, but when I said, 'Are you afraid of getting emotionally close to her?' Laura absolutely dissolved into tears. She was fearful of getting attached to this little girl because she knew that she was going to die and she wanted to protect herself from the pain of having to say goodbye to this baby. By this time Pete was in tears too and they cried together. We kept with it for a while and had the following dialogue:
>
> > Chloe: After you have died and Pete talks to your children about you, telling them stories about their mum as they are growing up, will he be able to tell the same stories to your little daughter as he can to your older one?
> >
> > Laura: No, he won't be able to.
> >
> > Chloe: So is there something you can do that actually will help him to tell the same story? What stories would you like to tell?

That set them off, and it was really nice. I just sat back and listened to them telling each other about the stories that Pete would tell and the stories Laura would like him to tell.

When someone in a family faces terminal illness, bereavement and grief work can sometimes start before death. It may have been very difficult for Laura to confront her prognosis, yet working through the pain of knowing the truth opened a channel of communication to the benefit of all the family members. Laura was a patient, and she was dying, but in sharing the stories to tell the children she was still a mother and a spouse in the here and now. She was living her dying.

Acknowledgements

Text extracts from Mayne, M., *The Enduring Melody*, Darton, Longman and Todd, London, UK, Copyright © 2006, reproduced with permission from Darton, Longman and Todd publishers.

References

Mayne, M. 2006. *The Enduring Melody*. London: Darton, Longman & Todd.

Vess, J. D., Moreland, J. R. and Schwebel, A. I. 1985. An empirical assessment of the effects of cancer on family role functioning. Journal of Psychosocial Oncology, 3, 1–16.

Vess, J. D., Moreland, J. R., Schwebel, A. I. and Kraut, E. 1988. Psychosocial needs of cancer patients: learning from patients and their spouses. Journal of Psychosocial Oncology, 6, 31–51.

Chapter 12

Chaplaincy and spiritual care

For centuries there has been a historical awareness of the connection between health and spiritual well-being. Indeed, much early medical practice, research, and care in the Western World was promoted within monasteries and executed by monks and nuns. As medicine developed, the spiritual and religious ethos was maintained and still has a special moral and ethical impact on the practice and structures of hospitals and other medical establishments. While in some ways this impact is reducing, it is still widely considered of great importance, especially in the realm of research ethics and the pastoral care of patients in active treatment. One of the signs of the historic importance of spirituality, whether it is widely recognised or not, is that almost all hospitals and hospices have chapels or quiet rooms on the premises, to provide a place where people can be still to pray or think, and where worship can be conducted.

Before developing this topic of chaplaincy and spiritual care, we want to remind the reader of our understanding of spirituality as an innate sense of another dimension to which we can aspire. It involves awareness of emotions, of bodily experiences, of what one is doing in this world, and how one is experiencing the world. It is discovered in relationships, in meeting people, in celebration, and in prayer. Spirituality expresses itself for good or evil uniquely in every person. It may bring a sense of integration, of wholeness, of unity, of harmony, of peace, of love, or their opposites. Religion can be an expression of spirituality, but it is not automatically so. We remind the reader of our metaphor 'Spirituality is the hand; religion is the glove which fits it'. Each helps to define the other; fitting may be a difficulty and gloves can be changed or discarded, but we agree with Stoter (1995 p. 7), who considers that spirituality is a universal capacity within the human race, which people may choose to develop or not.

The role of the chaplain

The role of the chaplain is clearly established in the National Health Service and is particularly strong in hospices, where holistic care is given pre-eminence. The chaplain is often a full-time or part-time member of staff who is called upon to serve as a focus and the lead practitioner of spiritual care for the well-being, not only of patients, but also of members of staff and volunteers. While not given any hierarchical status or rank, the chaplain is a member of the multi-disciplinary team, subject to contracts and disciplines, but is generally given freedom of access that is often denied to others. The chaplain is expected to be available to all on the site regardless of status or role and is often assisted by ministers of various Christian denominations and, in the multicultural society of today, by leaders of other faiths. Their role is generally welcomed, often for more than religious reasons.

Chaplains normally receive training, but they frequently develop their own style and spiritual outlook on their work, calling upon their personal spiritual background and experience and the traditions and writings over the centuries. James, a priest to whom we talked, shared

> *I like to think of my ministry as a two-legged sacrament. I visit the sick as a physical expression of God's love, remembering God is already there, and I wear clerical dress to emphasise this. As a chaplain you need to be rooted in prayer, which can be hard work sometimes. Personal prayer is the root of your personal and spiritual relationship with the person who is ill.*

When visiting the sick, the chaplain may come as a friend, but is more than that. In their pastoral role they help the patient to discover their spirituality and, where relevant, can take the prayer life and the liturgical life of the faith to their bedside. This is why James says that he will always ask the person: 'Shall I pray for you?'. If they agree he will pray with them. If not, he offers to hold them in his own prayers.

Using a slightly different metaphor, Alice likes to feel that she 'brings the Christ-light' to her work.

> *I go to the patient as a Christian minister; therefore I take that Christ-light to them. But that doesn't mean to say I talk about Christ. Hopefully the Christ-light shines on where they need to be looking. It's like going to somebody with a searchlight on your head, and helping them to see what they need to look at in their dark reality.*

Alice's reflections bring to the fore how religious care should not be forced upon the patient; she does not always talk about Christ. She considers it essential that the patient's autonomy is not challenged. Prayer still can be important, as Eve explains.

> *More people pray than you realise. They will say, 'I'm not religious, but I pray every night.' So generally at the end of a conversation, if there's been any mention at all of God, I'll say, 'May I pray with you?' or 'Would you like me to pray for you in the chapel or here or at a service?'. Nearly always they want*

me to pray with them. I take their hand and reflect to God on what they said, giving thanks—because I think that's what people are doing in a way, they're giving thanks for what is good. Acknowledging the uncertainty of the present and praying for hope and strength to cope with the future. I'm sure there are more people I could pray with than I actually have the nerve to, because I'm so anxious about imposing it on someone.

That both James and Eve offer to pray with and for patients shows how important this support can be and so too can holding hands with people who are very ill or dying. It conveys a deep sense of being accompanied, of not being alone.

One of us, recovering from major surgery, had this experience in the intensive care unit. Throughout the night following the operation, a male nurse did not move from the bedside and held the patient's hand and occasionally stroked it. It conveyed a profound sense not only of companionship, but even in the semi-conscious state, also a sense of assurance and hope.

Something so simple and direct seemed a sign of healing, with powerful and positive spiritual impact.

Caution not to impose

Chaplaincy and religious care have moved a long way from the Victorian practice of hurrying to say and do the important and right things to 'save the patient's soul'. Nowadays, theological discussions and sacramental life are brought in only when the patient asks for them or drops a hint. Often it will be a member of the nursing staff who will act as an intermediary, asking when they feel it appropriate 'Would you like to see the chaplain?'. This again stresses the patient's autonomy, making it easier for the patient to say 'No, thank you' than it would be to reject a chaplain standing in front of them.

Chaplains' caution not to impose prayer or overt religion is probably a mark of our secular times, but also of respect for differences of outlook. James, Alice, and Eve, without forcing anything upon anyone, are still keen to open a door and offer religious and spiritual care. James shared the following recollections:

I would pray for the patients all the time, as far as possible, but I wouldn't normally pray overtly with them, unless they ask. There's always a danger of praying at people, addressing them but pretending you're talking to God, using prayer to say things you want them to hear. That's naughty! They're on a journey out of this life, out of this world, and I'd like to do all I can as God's agent to reassure them of His love and forgiveness and hear their confession if that's appropriate, but often it may not be, because they aren't used to that kind of thing.

We may recall Louis (see Chapter 9, 'Flexibility in approach and response'), a doctor involved in medical training, sending medical students out to ask patients about their religion or spirituality. He further commented:

When patients were asked 'Would you like to speak to the hospital chaplain?' some patients replied 'Oh no, I won't bother him'. And they similarly ignored hints about contacting their own church: 'Oh, I think they know I'm here, I had a card from them'. If they then were asked: 'Has anyone been to visit?' they would say, 'Well no, but I don't like to bother them'. And yet, when invited by the students to talk about this topic, it seemed quite spontaneous to get the healing processes activated.

Patients not wanting to bother the chaplain or local vicar who 'knows' are perhaps speaking volumes about their wish to be visited or their anxiety about what might happen. If they know the chaplain is available, they can make up their own minds without pressure. We feel therefore that the initiative to inform patients about the chaplain's availability should rest with the nurses or other staff members who act as gatekeepers for the chaplaincy. This role is important because patients and their families may feel unsure about what is on offer, expected of them, or what would be the consequences. It is therefore vital that the chaplain has good relationships with other members of staff.

Spiritual care as giving meaning

As we have already noted, to suffer major illness has a profound impact on how people make sense of their lives. For some it brings fresh understanding, new meanings, but for others quite the opposite occurs: the meanings and directions they had are disrupted or lost. Neimeyer (2011), an American psychologist working with loss and grief, sees the core of his work as helping people make sense and find meaning in their shattered lives at practical, relational, and spiritual levels. Profound questions can be aroused, which challenge the bereaved: 'Why and how did he die?', 'How does that leave me to live the rest of my life?', 'If God is loving, why did he let this happen?'. These are important and pervasive questions. How or whether they are considered will influence the impact of the loss and what the sufferer will become in the future.

We see Eve, a hospital chaplain, putting this idea to work when she seeks people's narratives. She believes that the most useful thing she can do with people who are dying is to listen to their stories. She helps them to remember what was, without being false, and to find meaning in the telling, as so often these stories have a beginning, a middle, and an end. They are often about patients' sense of self, value, purpose, reparation, and completion in the process of letting go; indeed, their spiritual state. Eve says:

> I encourage people to talk about the significant things that have changed them and have made them who they are. I think people can find real healing and letting go in this, because if our story is complete then it's easier to let go, and because what we struggle with the most is that our life has no purpose, that we have just come about by accident.
>
> For people who have no faith—and a lot of people have no faith—I try to help them see their life had meaning and purpose through remembering and reflecting on what they enjoyed, what has been good—the garden, the cats, the family, the friends, the war experience.
>
> It's important that people can say what's happened, even the bad things. There's a sense of discovery, something that has come into focus through the illness. Although they knew that they were loved (or hoping they were), seeing the attentiveness of a family, all the letters that friends write helps them to believe it; they have something concrete to show. People don't often say, 'Now I'm ready to die because…', but there's a sense of that which allows them peacefulness, or the capacity to let go. That's important.
>
> Sometimes I want patients to know how privileged I've felt to listen to their story. People will draw their own meanings, but we can make them feel valued and significant by listening and then reflecting that. Whatever people's beliefs and expectations, I would want them to have such a sense of completion. In fact people feel (and are?) more special than ever because they're going to die and, partly because of their memories and all that's happened to them, we're drawing this story to a close—as complete as it can be—and we try to make it a good ending for them, whatever that may be.

Talking about who they have been seems to allow patients to touch again the feelings and the significance and purpose of their life. It opens up the kaleidoscope of all the facets of their personality rather than limiting it just to the illness or the fact that they are dying. Part of what is important for some patients is to have a sense that their living was worth the living and that they will have made a mark in some way. Sometimes it is quite difficult to know what kind of mark they have made and we can help them to recognise its reality.

Regrets and reparation

Out of this kind of review it may appear that a task needs to be done, something needs to happen or take place, some kind of reparation or completion to be undertaken. Chloe told the story of her work with Gilbert, who knew he was dying and wanted to come clean about the upset he had caused to his first wife. His sense of guilt skewed for him the meaning and significance of his life.

> *Gilbert was very happy with his second wife, but the reason he had married a second time was because he had an affair with this woman while he was still married to his first wife. Towards the end of his life we had a conversation about who would be sad about him dying. He said, 'There's my first wife, and I don't know whether she would be sad'. Talking about what she might be feeling, he was left with the idea that she might be very angry still with him about what had happened because he had been very deceitful and he knew that she'd been very hurt, but at the time all he had wanted was to satisfy his own desires.*
>
> *We talked about whether there was a way of making reparation for that and whether there was something that he needed to do or say. He hadn't been in contact with his first wife for a long time, but he knew where she was. He wrote her a letter in which he didn't use the word 'forgiveness' but he said how sorry he was. At the time of the divorce proceedings it had all been very acrimonious, and knowing he was dying it was enormously important for Gilbert to be able to acknowledge that he had hurt someone very badly and that he was responsible and culpable for that.*
>
> *We talked about what would happen if he didn't get a reply and why was he doing this? Did he want to die with a clean slate? It wasn't about that. He was really sorry, and although things might not have been different, as he had been enormously happy with the second wife and didn't want to reduce the value of that, he was still aware that there was a bit in the middle where his behaviour was cruel and took no account of what it might have been like for his first wife.*

Chloe helped Gilbert to explore his guilt. He acknowledged the hurt of his first wife and her possible residual anger without taking anything away from his happy second marriage. He explored how to clear it up and make reparation for what had happened, independently of whether his first wife would be able to respond or not. For some, writing a letter is too big a thing to do. By helping them to express what they really want to say, the carer can help to simplify the stories patients tell themselves at the cost of huge emotional energy. The bottom line is often 'I love you', 'I really care about you', or 'I'm sorry'.

Gary Collins suggests that guilt is the point where religion and psychology most often meet (2007, p. 178), it can therefore be the cause of much suffering spiritually and psychologically. People express guilt in all sorts of ways. They can feel it as a burden, shame, or embarrassment. Some have the feeling of being convicted, ugly, and unclean. Others experience a deep sense of regret and responsibility for wrongdoing. For others still it can be rather vague, as in

'If only…'. Guilt cannot be taken at face value. It is important to explore guilt feelings and be realistic about what can be done about them. There is no magic way of saying 'I'm sorry' so that all is cleared and well for everyone.

When people are overseeing their whole life, they face issues that have made a difference for them and for others and cannot simply be waved away with words. Alice reports:

> One can seek forgiveness from a higher being; one can also seek forgiveness from somebody else, as with patients who have perhaps been estranged from a son or a daughter, and they are longing before they die for that person to visit. But there is also forgiveness of self, which can be the hardest bit.

We all have things in our lives that we would rather not have, that bit of our life that we hide from and we may be cross with ourselves for having done. Coming to terms with it is important for us all.

Acceptance of another person who has wronged one, or acceptance of one-self for our weaknesses or failures is important and can sometimes be the forerunner of forgiveness. However, that process may be a step too far. Ritual forgiveness through religious absolution where there is genuine regret and a desire to move forward may be a valuable aid to a new freedom from a sense of failure or guilt. It does not have to be sacramental but it has to include an authority either from God or a person of recognisable spirituality and wisdom. The chaplain can be the medium of such release.

Needs, spiritual and/or religious

These days it is not uncommon to confuse religious convictions with spirit-uality, and the difference of role between chaplain and therapist can also be blurred. In these confusions it is easy to overlook the value of the specifically religious content of chaplaincy, however this is presented. In palliative care it is generally recognised that spiritual care is the role of all the members of the multidisciplinary team. All have conversations helping patients and families make sense of their experience and their life as they approach death and are open to address questions and issues arising around that. It is therefore impor-tant to distinguish between spiritual care, which is the responsibility of all, and religious care which is more specifically the role of the chaplain.

However, although different, the roles of chaplain and therapist share some similarities, the most central being patient-centredness, which runs through the whole of the multidisciplinary team. Even so, there can still be a grey area, as one of us has experienced working as both a chaplaincy volunteer and a counsellor in the same specialist palliative care unit. The experience in distinguishing between these roles was one of clarity of purpose and boundaries. As a chaplaincy volunteer, the encounter had an open agenda; the only thing on offer was quality of presence and loving care. There was no certainty that there would be a conversation at all, and if there was, where it would go or how long it would take. As a counsellor her quality of presence was set in a contractual arrangement with clients to meet at regular intervals to achieve a mutually agreed goal. Conversations were focussed and there was a regular review in terms of meeting the set goals and how to improve this. Even though goals could be adapted or new ones could be brought in, there was a clear beginning, a middle, and an end to the counselling relationship.

Chris, once a chaplain, became a counsellor in the health sector. He was asked how he differentiated these roles. As a chaplain in a mental health hospital he used means similar to those of a counsellor to try to find ways to connect with patients and help them worship and/or express and explore parts of themselves and their faith. Over time Chris developed a growing interest in the patient's autonomous perspective and he perceived that his role as a representative of the church became an obstacle in this:

> *My problem with being a chaplain perhaps was that I was supposed to be leading the worship, giving the ideas out all the time, and I found that was no longer something I wanted to do. I wanted to find out what the patients' ideas were and tune into them, free to think about the words of a hymn, rather than them being told what this means.*
>
> *As a counsellor, my first aim is that people find ways to help themselves so that they become more autonomous. I think that is the job of the therapist. On the spiritual level, it's almost unspoken. When I'm with a patient or a client, I try to go beyond the superficial hoping to establish connectedness which may lead to that level 'beyond', and when it does, it's powerful and helpful. I think our job as a counsellor and as a spiritual carer is to recognise people's spirituality and help them to find it and to deepen it.*

This chaplain had, as he said, a problem that sheds light on a common confusion in our secular society about the nature and form of worship. Many still consider that worship depends fundamentally on the input of the leader, without taking seriously the ideas and presumptions of the members of the congregation and giving them value. The chaplain's role therefore can appear narrowly directive rather than what we believe it should be: that of companion, guide, or mentor in spiritual and religious things.

Many lay people do not understand the role of the chaplain. This reflects their general confusion about religion as their grasp depends on where they are in matters of faith. It can be that they have never heard of spirituality or it could be that they have as deep a conviction about learned religious truths as the chaplain. Religious teaching may be a means to personal growth and search for meaning. One cannot presume to know where one is in relation to the patient's background and beliefs. One has to discover it as one goes along. Sometimes a chance remark can set the ball rolling. Alice gives a vivid example:

> I went into one of the single rooms where Eileen, a new lady, had been admitted. She was very polite. Her husband was there and she said, 'Well I'm afraid I'm not religious' and then said, 'Do you know I've always regretted not being baptised'. So I just said, 'Well it's never too late', and moved on. But the next time I went back, she said, 'Did you mean what you said the other day about being baptised?' This was her way of starting to look at her relationship with a higher being. It took a little while, but eventually I was privileged to be able to baptise her.
>
> This is a very short example of a chance remark leading on to something else which could easily have been overlooked. I could have said, 'Oh that's fine, I'm not just here for the religious people'. But a throwaway remark took her gradually towards baptism and thinking what baptism meant, thinking about those things she needed forgiveness for and, in a way, preparing for her death.
>
> Eileen's husband couldn't cope with the fact that she was thinking about anything to do with God. He would have preferred to be anywhere else but in that chapel, but she wanted him there so he sat and held her hand. He looked incredibly uncomfortable through the whole process, but he ended up in tears. It had been wonderfully moving for him.

Had Alice been defensive about affirming her role as a chaplain to everyone in the hospice she might not have opened a door for Eileen. So often what makes a difference is saying or doing the right thing at the right time, often unaware. This situation highlights the importance of spontaneity. Yet, at other times the spontaneous response will not be the right one. As Jane, the doctor who used the 'polyfilla in a cup' metaphor said, 'When talking to people who are dying, you never know whether what you are going to say will be very right or very wrong'. It demands fine-tuning and flexibility on the part of the carer.

Furthermore, we cannot fully know the value of the encounter, except on some rare occasions where those concerned are left with a sense of wonder at the depth and mutual nourishment from what has happened. However, it is not so much what is said or not said—it is what the chaplain is, and shows. In it God may be revealed or not, or a door to the spiritual dimension opened or closed. Any conversation can convey deeper things than may first appear. The role and privilege of the chaplain is to help patients and their loved ones to recognise this discovery and its growth potential, by linking it with their own life-tested and personal spirituality.

Overlap of roles

Because we cannot separate out a patient's concerns, there can be an overlap of roles in the care for the chronic and terminally ill. Dame Cicely Saunders introduced the concept of total pain—physical, psychological, and spiritual. She warned clinicians in palliative care that their focus may often be on the pain rather than on the person. Alleviating suffering as best we can is the goal of holistic care. Sometimes a physical issue such as pain—which may also be social or psychological pain—must take precedence in order to free space for spiritual care. Alice commented:

> *We are whole people, and I think although we are there to deal with the spiritual, we may be overlapping in other areas. We may come across social or family problems that we can help the patient to deal with. In a similar way we may touch on psychological aspects and help them with that. In the same way other carers will touch on the spiritual life when they are looking after patients. But if somebody is in physical pain, they are going to tense up and they tend to make the pain worse by doing that.*

Spiritual care, as said earlier, is the remit of every member of the multidisciplinary team. We feel that the fundamental difference between religious and spiritual care resides in the nature of the relationship. The chaplain comes as a representative of a religious community and God, with love for and recognition of the patient's uniqueness, value, and importance, not only to himself, his family and circle of friends, but also to God. The dimensions of the relationship are thus different, but the results—growth and peace for the patient—we hope and trust are the same.

Whether religious or not, people have spiritual needs. As a hospital chaplain Eve thinks it would be lovely if there could be a 'spiritual friend' throughout the journey; somebody who is there not to monitor physical symptoms but to express the importance of those deep spiritual things and to support the patient and those involved emotionally, starting as soon as the early stages of the illness. She says:

> *So often there are communication problems between people; you hear things that aren't being said. Patients say 'I could say this' and I think 'You should be saying this to your family', but they think it would upset their family. I try to visit when the family is there, encouraging them to talk about funerals, or decisions, or things that patients or families would wish*

for. But sometimes patients don't have as much time as they expect and things get in the way.

Sadly many patients go through the whole illness process choosing not to get information about their condition or not to assimilate what is going on. They are not always given the right information about their chances to live and die, and by the time they are facing their death their timeframe is very short and does not allow sufficient opportunity for things to be completed. This can be overwhelming and chaplains and spiritual carers in the hospital or hospice setting share the concern of therapists that they are often called in at the last minute and have to resort to crisis intervention. We favour a longer-term approach where possible; this would be more helpful and fulfilling towards bringing peace and that special sense of completion.

Death and dying

One area where chaplains and clergy in general are deemed to have particular knowledge is around what happens to the dying person after death. The factual answers of course are particularly unclear. However, Eve commented:

When people are dying they often call us as chaplains: even if they are not religious, they think that is what their mother or father would have wanted.

There are some written prayers like 'Go forth upon thy journey, O Christian soul', which are wonderful and deeply historical prayers which have been prayed with people for many years.

Go forth upon they journey from this world, O Christian soul,
In the love of God the Father who created you;
In the mercy of Jesus Christ who redeemed you;
In the power of the Holy Spirit who strengthens you;
May the heavenly host sustain you,
The company of heaven enfold you,
And in communion with all the faithful,
May you dwell this day in peace.

Traditional Roman prayer

The chaplain can bear witness to the Christian hope of resurrection, but still be very unclear about what that means in practice. Similarly chaplains of other faiths will seek to bring understanding about what they believe might happen after death to their adherents. It becomes a matter of shared faith and hope: the chaplain's commitment to those dimensions encourages others; they also give a framework to the fundamentals of being a person.

The chaplain is also possibly in a privileged position when it comes to certain elements of grief. When the patient has been resident in a hospice for a time, a relationship may have been built up between that patient and his family and the chaplaincy, which leads sometimes to a request for the chaplain to take the funeral. This in turn could enable a continuing link between the family and those responsible for bereavement care in the hospice, which, in the context of an established relationship, can be a considerable help to the bereaved family for as long as is necessary—a gift rarely available in society as a whole.

Where the family experience a sense of guilt over their relief that a person has passed away after a long and painful dying, the chaplain may offer a particular reassurance and succour helping them to understand their feelings. It is relief from suffering for the patient and for the family as well, as the huge strain of watching someone die by the inch is lifted. This was the case for Sara.

Sara, aged 43, took five months to die from advanced Hodgkin's disease. At the end, she was blind, deaf, and weighing 65 pounds. She was like a living skeleton. At her death there was at first genuine thanksgiving. Subsequently, a sense of guilt set in about those feelings. It was the parish priest who was able to absolve some members of the family from that sense of guilt over their new freedom, and able to point them to the truths of their love and their long-term care for Sara, and her certain wish that they should commit themselves to a new life without her.

Amidst the natural sense of loss and grief, when suffering ceases, relief and freedom can be welcomed for the patient and the family. Everything possible has been done and a new life—in Christian terms—opens up for all the participants in that painful drama.

References

Collins, G. R. 2007. *Christian Counselling: A Comprehensive Guide, 3rd edn.* Nashville: Thomas Nelson.

Neimeyer, R. A. and Sands, D. C. 2011. Meaning reconstruction in bereavement. From principles to practice. In: Neimeyer, R. A., Harris, D. L., Winokuer, H. R. and **Thornton, G. F.** (eds.), *Grief and Bereavement in Contemporary Society. Bridging Research and Practice.* New York: Routledge, p. 9–22.

Stoter, D. 1995. *Spiritual Aspects of Health Care.* London: Mosby.

Part 4

Boundaries and resources

Chapter 13

Blurred boundaries

The personal and intimate nature of the relationship between a professional carer and patient and the poignancy of the potentially terminal outcome of an illness can challenge the way carers and therapists manage boundaries. There is an emotional cost to working with the chronically and terminally ill, which needs attention. The following stories and reflections highlight a number of boundary issues that came up in the interviews.

Expectations and projections

Reading through the narratives it is evident that the therapist, the spiritual carer, the nurse, the doctor, the social worker, the volunteer, the friend, and the family all counsel. What is the difference between them? In search of best practice, professions clarify what they offer; but what about the patient's expectation?

One of us, having worked for more than seven years in palliative care, has been struck by how little patients discriminated between who offers what. Patients do not wait until the doctor's visit to ask about the itch that came up in the night, they will ask the first person they see and they will also ask any person who passes by for a drink, for help with the pillows, or even to go to the lavatory. They have questions, feel sick, are anxious about their families, have administrative or financial worries, struggle to make sense of the disruption in their lives, feel guilty, appreciate the care and pain relief; all of this colours how they are and what they may or may not want to talk about, when and to whom. Yet all professionals have their specialities and competences, things they can and cannot do, not least according to health and safety regulations. How can we clarify and negotiate the patient's expectations in the light of the professional's offering? How do we affirm the family carers' role in relation to the professionals coming from outside without diminishing their responsibilities and commitment?

Intrigued, we held a small poll, asking ourselves and others what we had expected as patients. The consultant's visit brought hope and fear: relief that one might be discharged from hospital, anxiety about the latest results, information discussing the treatment, but also hope that the consultant might be pleased with how the patient was doing. The nurse is seen as a friend, encouraging and welcoming, as a performer of nursing acts or even a servant. There can be a more intimate relationship with the night nurse, who is reassuring and may help the patient through a difficult patch. Allied health professions can be associated with pain and struggle, as in rehabilitation physiotherapy, or with relaxation and well-being, as in aromatherapy and massage. The visit of a psychotherapist arouses gratitude or perhaps concern: 'She's come to sort me out' or anxiety and resistance: 'Maybe he thinks I'm not coping or going a little mad'. On the other hand, the visit of a chaplain can be challenging or surprising: 'Why has he come?'. If one is offered communion or another sacrament the visit might match an expectation or lead to a sense of embarrassment, feeling that 'My religion is a private affair and I don't want it identified in public'.

Whether positive or negative, apprehensive or welcoming, broad or narrow, expectations condition what the patient can hear and accept. We need to take these expectations into account, making space for them and clarifying what we have to offer accordingly. Clothing has an effect: a stethoscope can make the patient and family anxious, curious and often rather subdued; badges, if they can be seen, are scrutinised to try and work out who they are talking to. Some people may feel relieved to keep it as a friendly visit when they see the chaplain's clerical collar, while others will also want to feel carried by his prayer because they feel that they cannot or are not worthy to offer it themselves. We doubt, however, that patients with no hospital background are aware of the differences in the blouses or other indicators of status or role worn by nurses, volunteers, and allied professionals, not to mention social workers and psychotherapists, who have no dress code.

Since the experiment with Pavlov's dog in 1904, psychological research has shown much evidence of how the expectations of the hearer are fundamental to their understanding of what is going on. This raises issues that are worth a research project, especially if we recognise how the effect of therapy and care depends on the match between what is offered and what is expected. We cannot ignore the baggage of past experience, which conditions our response to things and people, for instance the fear of the unknown and the unfamiliar, a sense of isolation and loneliness, or the questions 'What have I done to deserve this?' and 'Now I'm here, what is expected of me?'.

It takes professional competence to be aware of people's expectations and work with them, but personal sensitivity must also be used in addressing these issues. Many doctors say that they are better doctors for having had the experience of being a patient.

A friend told us that never, in his fifteen years of practice as a surgeon, had he realised how frightening medical instruments are; he experienced a huge sense of vulnerability and fear when they were pushed up his nose. Having his polyps removed has changed his practice, and now he always takes time to comfort people before intervening.

Research and experience in psychotherapy stress the importance of defining the boundaries with the client. Matters of confidentiality, time, duration, and cost of the sessions need to be clarified. More than just agreeing on practical issues, this clarity is about sharing power in the relationship, having a shared understanding of what the problem is, how it is perceived, how it will be tackled, and about what is expected by both the therapist and the client. In psychotherapy there is an additional check of whether client and therapist feel comfortable with each other. Medical and nursing conditions do not usually leave room for the latter, but one can always take the time to recognise issues of perception and expectation and try to clarify them in a shared understanding.

Shared responsibility

Carers—whether professionals, volunteers or family members—offer the patient the presence and security of having somebody there. They are people who are prepared to give of themselves. Professionals make available their expertise as nurse, therapist, or doctor, and also share with the patient some of their personal qualities, such as attention, spirituality, humour, and their inner being. The volunteer gives of their time and of their personal qualities too. The relative or friend gives of their love, faithfulness and commitment.

There will be some people with whom carers fail because there is nothing more that they have to offer, or because the patient cannot cooperate or does not want to explore their feelings—and that is their right. If one of us had cancer we might decide that we do not want radiotherapy. The doctor might promise a 99.9 % chance that the tumour will go if we have radiotherapy, but whether we have it or not is ultimately our choice. Rabinovitch (2007) talked with her doctor about the cost of treatment, wondering whether she would live any longer because of it. Apart from the financial implications, patients are not always aware of the cost of travelling to and from the hospital for treatment—in wear and tear, discomfort, and indeed the amount of time involved. As all treatments can fail or have difficult side effects, there remains the question of the use of time when life may be short.

Patients are not always aware that they have a choice. Their attitude depends on the information available to them and on how they perceive the caregiver.

One of us remembers talking to a patient whose course of chemotherapy had been interrupted because her blood count levels and markers were critical. She was not feeling well, and when asked what she would really like she said: 'I trust my doctor. If he thinks it's right to have more chemotherapy, I'll go for it.' She did not even dare to ask what the consequences were.

Looking up to the doctor, this patient did not take part in the decision. The idea that there was an option had not even occurred to her. Heyse-Moore (2009, pp. 84–85) indicates this is a recurring phenomenon. Most patients follow their doctor's advice because they believe it will increase their chances of survival. They struggle with taking responsibility for their illness and its management and do not feel able to make the technical decision through their lack of knowledge or experience. After all, they think, the doctor knows best and many doctors expect compliance with their advice.

The responsibilities of the professional working with the chronically ill or dying person can be very exacting, especially when there is likely to be a strong sense of dependence. The recognition that 'after all they are the professionals' will have strong influence over the patient or client, however carefully guidance and care are delivered. The extent of responsibility is variable according to the circumstances, but we consider that the focus should be on the patients and responsibility *towards* them rather than in a direct sense of responsibility *for* them. The professional will be working within frames of reference and will be answerable to their employer or professional body but should not take responsibility from the patient or their immediate relatives, who must be the final arbiters.

It can be very difficult for some patients to give themselves the choice. Some might even feel more secure if the doctor or the nurse or anybody else makes these difficult decisions for them. Our experience as patients has been that feeling part of the decision-making was healing. A trusting relationship, in which the options and their possible consequences and the doctor's recommendation were made explicit, helped us feel part of what was happening. This raised our morale as well as our physical well-being and progress.

Not all healthcare professionals feel comfortable in giving 'their' patients power. This may be due to the fact that they may not have been trained in power-sharing or because they choose to keep a distance as part of their emotional self-protection against the pressures of the work. Moreover, to be successful, a shared partnership between doctor and patient needs to be put in place from the very first meeting. Trusting and getting to know each other in the intimate way illness may demand takes time, and this may be a major professional challenge in overworked environments.

Individual and institution

It will be clear from the stories in this book that professional carers have to contend with personal and organisational boundaries. Nobody employed by a hospital or hospice can disassociate themselves from the patients' and the carers' expectations of the institution and, vice versa, from the institutions' expectations and plans for patients and carers. We have noted how organisational realities can influence or even short-circuit the encounter; a number of challenges can also arise from the possible (mis)match of individual and institution.

Has a junior doctor or a registrar the same weight as a consultant? We know of patients who have been far more sensitive to how attractive their doctor was than to his rank! Do doctors' perceptions of their position in their organisation affect how they relate to patients and staff? A friend who was a patient of a highly respected academic felt that his interest in her went no further than seeing her as an interesting research subject.

The wider question of the capacity in which carers work has implications for the perceptions and expectations of patients and carers. It also has an impact on the carer's accountability in the carer–patient relationship. This affects both professional and lay carers. A therapist who is external to an organisation can bring a different perspective. Independent of the institution, the client is the focus and the external therapist may help the patient to take responsibility for themselves, both in and outside the medical environment. Boundary issues here have to do with personal involvement and cost to the therapist of losing someone they have grown close to.

Therapists and doctors working in a hospice, a hospital, or a paramedical organisation on the other hand can find themselves facing institutional obligations that compete for the time and support they can offer a client or a family. The dual responsibility to the patient and the institution can lead to ethical dilemmas. In times of limited resources, this can be highlighted in the choice of drugs to be used in a particular case, with cheaper, less beneficial ones used in preference to the better but more expensive ones. An inbuilt duty and control mechanism in institutions tends to limit the personal scope for action. Issues of confidentiality and boundaries can arise. For the clinical staff within an institution, the primary focus should be 'coping with' the implications and consequences of the illness and harnessing the patient's strengths and resources to do so.

Information and self-disclosure

Some interviewees found that their nursing background and knowledge of treatment could effectively be brought into their conversations with patients, even though at the start they were hesitant to do so. They felt that as counsellors or chaplains they were in another profession and had left nursing behind. Sue reflected:

> *For some patients and clients, my knowledge of the process of the treatment was very useful. For some clients it wasn't, and I would never even go there nor even tell them. Others were fearful, wanted reassurance, or I suggested that the next time they were up at the hospital they would mention their query and check it out with the nurses or doctor. What made a difference to patients was the reassurance that they were not going mad, that this was all right and that they could regain control of their own life.*

Here again, there is no general rule. Ex-nurses or ex-doctors using their knowledge to reassure and encourage a patient in a counselling encounter are wary of being seen as replacing the direct link with the nursing and medical team. Yet they realise that in some cases their input can help patients and families to make the most of an upcoming encounter with their doctor or nurse, to whom they always refer.

> *In her work with patients facing life-altering illness, Rachel tried to help people be aware of what might be helpful to them, such as leaflets and information, but also emotional resources and parts of themselves that they can turn to when things are difficult. A former and long-retired nurse, she was very discreet about sharing medical knowledge in case it undermined the relationship between the patient and their doctors and nurses. However, by her manner, she tried to give encouragement and confidence so that each medical hurdle was successfully accepted and coped with. Rachel also recognised that by providing medical facts and knowledge, she could be in danger of avoiding her real task of helping the patients come to terms with their feelings.*

The issue of just how and how much of their personal experience should be revealed by the carer is related at its deepest level, not to supplying information, but to sharing something of humanity. Empathy, as we have considered, is crucial, providing intimacy, but also space between carer and patient, allowing for a deep understanding of the other's hopes and fears. By helping to reveal something of themselves, the carer can add a subtle support based on that common humanity and solidarity—we are all fearful, pain is ghastly, death is the great unknown. It is not a question of providing answers, but of sharing the struggle. The patient or client is helped to realise that as a human being they are not alone. As things ebb and flow in the course of the illness, patient and carer may recognise this deep companionship on the way, but also that they remain, in all the changes, vulnerable and exposed.

The challenge of visiting the dying

Two psychotherapists interviewed worked with terminally ill clients until they died. They had to make decisions about their line of conduct in these exceptional circumstances. Benedict made the following comment:

> *The point came when Arthur had to be hospitalised. His cancer ward was an ordeal of suffering, pain and appalling smells of suppurating wounds. He was full of tubes and his family was finding it very difficult to visit. From his sick bed, Arthur suggested that they bring me along, so they would feel stronger. It was a moving experience for me; it was a difficult one too.*
>
> *My task was not to spend too much time with them but to protect them and enable them to meet in a way that was neither overpowering for him nor overwhelming for them. We used to meet up beforehand, outside the hospital. It was a question of giving them strength to survive the physical ordeal as much as the emotionality of it. These visits happened four or five times.*

Similarly, Joanne had been working with Veronica, the diarist, for over three years when her client no longer had the energy to come to see her. This is when Joanne decided to end the professional part of their relationship. She visited Veronica in her home as 'a companion on the journey' and there would be no more paying. She writes about her experience towards the end of Veronica's life:

> *During the last week of her life I saw Veronica once. Each day I met her husband and her friend as they nursed her with McMillan nurses. I remember collecting the first prescription of morphine, being part of the 'case conference' with the GP in her home, and sitting by her an hour or two after she died, saying my goodbyes.*
>
> *At her funeral I read a story she wrote. I think of her every year at the anniversary. I remember the sand tray (as a Jungian therapist, Joanne used a sand tray as a medium to visualise and express feelings) and always the little black creature in the corner of the tray—I guess it was her fear. She would bring a summer iris, rolled up tight, and we would put it in water and during the session it would open out.*

It is notable how Benedict and Joanne, both individual therapists, became involved with their terminally ill client's family and friends towards the end. In both these cases it seemed a natural move, as if from journeying deeply with a dying client they became personally involved and felt a sense of responsibility to support the client's nearest and dearest in a way the client would have wanted.

Furthermore, such journeying with the client until the end may be a means of dealing with the therapist's own sense of loss. Joanne said how important making her goodbyes after Veronica's death and taking an active part in the funeral arrangements were for her. Rachel, on the other hand, felt bereft of a means of dealing with her residual grief when she decided not to go to a client's funeral. Deciding to stick to the clear boundary of her role as counsellor she denied herself a possible means of helping to work through her experience of loss.

Both Joanne's and Rachel's experiences remind us of the reciprocity that may come from a relationship between a counsellor and a client who is dying when they relate at depth and boundaries become blurred. Being there for another person is healing, not only for the one dying but for those around him. All are human and all share the burden of loss as well as the reality of our mortality. We wonder whether, when a client is embarking on the final stages of his life, in his dying or death, his presence may offer some healing to the counsellor that walks alongside him at that time.

References

Heyse-Moore, L. 2009. *Speaking of Dying. A Practical Guide to Using Counselling Skills in Palliative Care.* London and Philadelphia: Jessica Kingsley Publishers.

Rabinovitch, D. 2007. *Take Off Your Party Dress. When Life's Too Busy for Breast Cancer.* London: Pocket Books.

Chapter 14

A wealth of resources

Where do patients and carers find the strength and courage to live with dying? What nourishes and supports them? In this penultimate chapter we look more specifically at things that may help people when they are confronted with life-altering illness. Many of these suggestions have been highlighted in the stories we have already recounted and may seem repetitive. However, we feel that it is appropriate to summarise resources relating to questions implied in the title of this book *Life to be Lived*.

From being the subject of suffering to an observer of pain

Earlier we have described personal sources of strength such as values, attitudes, absorbing interests, prayer, and the solace of nature. These resources relate to ways in which the illness and the process of dying can be taken on board. Individuality is the key. How personal wells of strength can become a resource is strikingly described by Martin Laird (2006 pp. 106–107), who distinguishes physical pain from suffering. By the latter he means the stories people tell themselves about their pain. He gives an account of Elizabeth, who was struck down by an auto-immune disease that caused her great pain. When she fretted and fussed about the pain, it increased. In Laird's words, she suffered as a result of what her mind did with the pain. However, when she relaxed and accepted the pain, its impact on her was reduced. Elizabeth found that her thoughts about pain were worse than the pain itself. Gradually, with practice, Elizabeth was able to let go of her pain and she felt alive and aware. She moved from being the subject of suffering to an observer of pain.

Somehow suffering dramatises the pain and makes it harder to bear. Keating speaks of the 'afflictive emotions' by which people respond to the experience of pain. He distinguishes four upsetting emotions, or combinations of emotions, that we put into place to protect ourselves from pain. Firstly, he cites anger. Secondly, apathy which can present as pervasive boredom, bitterness or recurrent frustration. Thirdly, he mentions lust or the overweening desire for satisfaction whether physical, mental or spiritual to compensate for the intolerable loss. Fourthly he cites pride which may be experienced as self-rejection or self-inflation (Keating, 2003 pp. 23–24). Awareness of afflictive emotions can be a way of moving from being a victim of suffering to being a witness of pain.

Kabat-Zinn (1990, 2003) bases his 'Mindfulness' approach on learning to focus on the pain. Letting their breath flow into and out of the painful area, patients are invited to be aware of any pain without trying to change it. Surprisingly such mental activity reduces the pain rather than increasing it. Such thinking seems to cause some mental separation from it, so that patients are no longer fixated on the cause (Heyse-Moore, 2009 p. 67). As the patient's anxiety reduces, so does the pain. On the other hand, if we dwell on the pain, it seems to increase. Thus we can see the possibility that our awareness of a pressure point can be stronger than our emotional or physical distress: perhaps a case of mind over matter. Mindfulness has successfully relieved patients of chronic pain, both malignant and non-malignant. It is not a quick fix though, and people need to practice regularly to benefit.

Other resources to try and change the experience of pain are relaxation and visualisation (Ferrucci, 1982, Glouberman, 1989, Johnson, 1986). People are invited to imagine a comfortable and safe place and to notice what they see, hear, smell, and feel. The strength of the method lies in its association with images from the person's memory, thus enhancing the relaxation. Sometimes visualisation is extended to facilitate an encounter with a significant figure as a source of advice and wisdom, which can have a powerful effect. The Bristol Cancer Help Centre (Hayes *et al.*, 1990) has devised a care model using visualisation to imagine fighting the cancer cells as an invading force, and this, they have found, can boost a patient's immune system.

Professional and peer support

When people get stuck, counselling can help with releasing the loss, anger, and resentment that may be lingering. It is also a place where it is possible to explore how to negotiate boundaries, an important skill in dealing with issues of transition and conflicting expectations.

Therapists working with patient groups seek to provide a space and time for the group members to help and support each other. Jennifer runs a stress-reduction course for women with primary breast cancer. She organises so-called 'refresher groups', where patients who have participated in a course come back after a while to share their experiences. Meeting with breast cancer survivors proves very helpful to the patients. Their feelings and worries may be normalised by hearing 'survivors' tell of their struggles and how they have coped. She told the story of Maureen:

The Breast Care nurses who thought she needed some help with anxiety had referred Maureen, a woman in her thirties with a young child. I was not sure whether her anxiety was in response to a very pessimistic diagnosis or whether she was excessively anxious in her dealing with everyday life. She joined the relaxation group and found it really helpful, but the anxiety persisted. She asked if I could see her for counselling privately.

She had decided to go back to university. This was normalising, but caring for a child, while doing a university course and running a home, placed much on her plate, not to mention the overriding anxiety about her illness: Would she be well? Would she stay well? How long did she have? Would the cancer come back?

The GP put Maureen on antidepressants. It helped taking her off the bottom but she would get so anxious, she forgot everything. She just panicked. When Maureen came to a refresher session something very good happened to her. She had a chance to talk about her anxiety and other people said they had felt the same. She phoned me to say how helpful she had found that support, how she could really hear it and take it in.

When meeting people who have gone through similar ordeals, patients feel less alone. This does not mean that other people's solutions are necessarily right or welcome.

One of us remembers a woman being treated for breast cancer saying how fed up she was by the number of people inundating her with tips about books to read and diets to follow. She indeed welcomed the advice, but in the end she wanted to do this her way and felt the ever-so-well-meaning comments were an intrusion.

The peer group offers support and encouragement as well as realistic backing. It should not encourage avoidance by being too soft in reducing the power of the pressure rather than adjusting to it. Peer-group support focuses on specific themes, such as 'How you make the transition from being a patient'. The support can also be very practical. Chris, a counsellor in the occupational health centre of a hospital, ran a group for staff who had to suspend or end their work because of illness. They discussed matter-of-fact issues such as money and volunteering jobs that they could do while on sick leave. He remembered Maud, who had been working as a nurse until she was diagnosed with cancer. She was expected to live only a few more years.

I met Maud very early on after her diagnosis and she joined the group. In her fifties, she was motherly and dynamic. When the group talked about how unfairly they felt they had been treated by their employer, Maud was the one who would suggest doing something about it and the group tended to rely on her initiative.

Maud wanted to write a book to help children who were diagnosed with cancer. It was in part autobiographic. She used to bring chapters to the group members to read and give comments. Being involved in something creative was valuable. People in the group had each other's telephone numbers, so that they could make contact if they wanted to and some did. They began to socialise and meet up for coffee, which was brilliant because some had been very isolated and depressed.

Maud's book-writing was healing for her and for the group members who took part. The group empowered Maud's self-realisation in supporting her writing as much as she gave them a focus, something to which they could contribute from their experience and skills. We will see later how hands-on involvement of different kinds can be a healing resource.

Working in a specialist palliative care day unit we have been struck by patients' testimonies about how much they value coming in each week. Whilst their being away for the day offered relief for home carers, the day unit expanded the patient's experience of the world, which was restricted by the illness. Coming to the centre was for some the highlight of their week. They met a number of people, did unusual things, enjoyed a good meal and made friends with other patients.

A lady told us that she used to be shy and reserved. In this group she was very much the cheerleader. She said 'I had to become ill and come here to develop that side of me.'

Many day units offer a range of activities. Besides patients' health and condition being monitored during those weekly visits, they can try out a craft and go home with candles, cards, photographs, and special gifts they have made. They can also enjoy complementary therapies and 'look well, feel good' make-up and 'head-start', where women who have lost their hair through chemotherapy are taught different ways of wearing scarves and hats. Some patients have never experienced any of this before and it gives them a sense of being special.

Hands-on involvement

A number of patients facing (terminal) illness discover and enjoy qualities that they did not suspect in themselves and in people around them. Many come to value lunch clubs and other social groups for the first time. They may even learn to use a computer or practice arts and crafts. There is a wide range of possibilities provided by hospices and other volunteer organisations. With time and encouragement patients and carers may develop the courage to take up such opportunities to their great advantage.

Working with their hands can help people who have reached a stage of their life when other occupations are no longer possible. Such contributions can come in all sorts of ways: It might be quilting, needlework, photography, mosaic…Thus Mary, who did not know what to do with herself when she was in hospital, discovered a new craft, as Alice recalls:

> *Mary was a single lady who had given her life to her medical career and caring for her mum. We had the following conversation:*
>
> Mary: *The trouble is I get to about a quarter to ten in the morning and I think: 'What am I going to do all day?'*
>   *Mary was not used to that. She was used to being busy, busy.*
> Alice: *When you were busy at work and you thought about taking early retirement, apart from the travelling—which you can't do today, in a few weeks that may be different—what did you think you would like to be doing?*
> Mary: *Well, I like using my hands.*
>
> *She pointed out there were two books about basket making on her bed, which the specialist palliative care nurse had left because she does CBT (Cognitive Behavioural Therapy) with her.*
>
> Alice: *Oh, does that interest you?*
> Mary: *Yes, I think it does.*
> Alice: *Well, we could get some for you now if you would like.*
> Mary: *Yes*
> Alice: *I think if you would like to do it, I will go and find one of the occupational therapists. We have some simple baskets, which you do with plastic. They have already the uprights.*
>
> *I went down to the OT who, although she was almost going home, very kindly unlocked the cupboard and we brought a variety of baskets to Mary. The basket-making industry started there and then. She got absolutely hooked on it. She realised that she was doing something useful and productive.*
>
> *The next day she asked 'What happens to these baskets?' and was told the hospice sold them towards the unit's costs. I bought the very first one she did because it was just a nice reminder. There was something there about being valued. Mary was producing something. How many people would see that as a spiritual need? But Mary's self-esteem went up. She was depressed and she was coming out of it with the basket making.*

It was not until she took to basket making that Mary could fill the day. It was keeping her busy and prevented her getting lost in thought, sometimes very negative. Maud and Mary found an identity in their creativity and productivity. They ended up with something tangible of which they could be proud and which people could encourage them in.

Patients who have been busy can find it hard when suddenly they do not have the energy to do the things they used to. Their value seems to be withdrawn.

> *Joanne, an elderly therapist, confided how she feared that a day would come when she could not look after herself any more. She feared that if and when she ended up in a care home she would have less opportunity to meet people with whom to share at her level of experience and understanding.*

When mental and physical decline do not match, there can be real suffering for the person. Alice tells of a similar need:

> *Frederick had worked very hard running a business which had made a name. He said, 'You know what I was used to, some nights I didn't go to bed. If I had a deadline, I would be up half the night, or all night framing pictures. Now, all I do is sit around doing jigsaw puzzles.'*
>
> *That rang a bell. Yes it is fun to do a jigsaw puzzle, but not every day. Could he not be found something to do where he was producing something, where he could feel he was contributing?*

It can also happen that patients discover new things in themselves during treatment and after-care. Such was the case for Maureen, the anxious young woman who had found significant support in the relaxation group. Her therapist reports:

> *A while later Maureen had a placement in her professional training. They needed somebody to teach some relaxation, and she wondered whether it would be okay for her to do this. She contacted me about it and asked to use some of my handouts. She herself was now teaching relaxation. She had been the recipient of something healing for her, had taken it on board, and was now teaching relaxation to others.*
>
> *When we spoke next, Maureen hardly mentioned the anxiety. She was getting on with life, having moved from thinking she couldn't do something to being in a position where she was called upon to do it and did. It made her feel really good. Doing something she had never expected of herself, she had become instrumental in something happening. From being turned inward on her issues and her problems, feeling detached and isolated, she was opening out.*

Maureen had gone to the relaxation group looking for help with her anxieties. Working through her issues in this way had had a snowball effect. She could now pass the relaxation on by teaching it—as the wounded healer—but could also integrate the experience and use it in other areas of life in unexpected ways.

When their condition progresses and patients miss the physical strength to practise any form of hands-on involvement, finding something meaningful to fill the day can become more challenging, and they may suffer distressing intro-spection about what they have lost in their lives. Being read poetry or a novel can be uplifting and sustaining. As Siobhan suggested, some have the nerve, the courage, and creativity to work out what they can still do with some help. Such was the case of a French journalist who moved one of us greatly. He suffered a 'locked-in syndrome'—literally, locked inside himself—after a stroke. He could no longer move, eat, talk, or even breathe without assistance. The only move-ment he had left was the blinking of his left eye. He managed to dictate a book (Bauby, 2007) for somebody to transcribe by blinking for every letter.

Ways to express feelings and find new meaning

As we have seen, the search for meaning covers spiritual characteristics of con-nectedness to self, others, the environment and The Other, as well as seeking the value/purpose in life and making sense of the ordeal one is facing. Arthur (see Chapter 3, 'Inner turmoil') and Ella (see Chapter 4, 'The part of life one has not lived') are two of many patients in whom healing presents a movement towards rediscovering a sense of personhood and identity, even if it was dif-ferent to how they felt about themselves before the illness. Journaling, writing a dream story or a letter or describing life imprints can help in having those conversations with ourselves and through them finding a constructive, bear-able, and nourishing meaning for the loss.

The search for meaning may throw up many questions and maybe unearth hidden personal sources of strength. Thus Siobhan, a psychotherapist who has had personal experience of life-limiting illness, has found artwork helpful to herself and others in getting past their inhibitions and their fear of anger so as to access deeper levels of meaning. She told the story of her work with Lynn:

Lynn was a woman in her late forties who suffered from lupus. It was very limiting for her. She was very frail, and walked with elbow crutches. There was a resignation about her: 'There's nothing I can do, I've got to live with it'. She couldn't do writing or drawing because her hands were too bad or she didn't have the energy, even when we set something up where she could be quite com-fortable. But something did not quite match. She couldn't write, and yet she used to do the accounts for her parents.

One day we had newspaper on the floor, a thick brush and strong colour paints—red, blue, yellow, bright primary colours. She picked red and black, and started off with large movements, swearing whilst she was doing it. She was shocked and said, 'I don't like this. I don't like this.' Lynn was deeply religious and she held this belief that God doesn't like anger. We explored what was wrong with anger, reframing it as a God-given emotion: not the anger was the problem, but what we did with it.

Lynn gradually began to see that there was a role-reversal in her family. Although she was so disabled, she acted as the parent and her parents were very childlike. The more she realised how her parents had suppressed her, the more her anger kept coming up.

When Lynn's father died, it was a release for her. She moved on and her mother moved on too. The lupus was still life-limiting, but it did not restrict her so much. She found another way of doing things. She went to a watercolour class in the village with her mother. It was sad that her father died, but Lynn realised that he'd held her and her mother back.

Some patients tend to be unaware of the anger and grudge they hold deep within them. They focus firmly on moving on with or despite the illness. The key for Lynn was to accept herself without the steely, 'Oh well I've got this, I've got to get on with it!'. Once she put her mark on the paper, she was shocked by what transpired. Questioning the colours and shapes, where she put things, the way she did it, she realised she held a great deal of anger. Allowing those feelings to come to the surface enabled her to acknowledge her fear, pain, and hurt. She could then come to a healthier acceptance of her life and her illness, which freed energy to develop new and different interests.

Siobhan's sensitivity to anger stems from her personal history of having to give up nursing when she hurt her back. She shared:

It was extremely painful because nursing was my life. The first time I hurt my back I was in bed for nine weeks. That was eighteen years ago and then last year, I had to stop my counselling work too, because my back went completely. I couldn't walk. I couldn't drive, I couldn't stand, I couldn't go to the toilet, I couldn't do anything and I had to wait ten months for surgery.

The difference now is that I can accept myself as I am in a loving way, rather than with the seething anger. I haven't given up fighting, because everything is a fight, but I look out for what I can do rather than what I can't. I always used to battle with everything, and I find I'm still hanging on to the counselling centre. But I look back now and think it's absolutely absurd to battle with that. All the energy and the time and emotions wasted! There's room for other possibilities and they're often better.

Writing and deep relaxation have helped me deal with the physical pain. Visualisation was the best one for me, especially of moving water, but also breathing—in for five and out for seven beats—and meditation. My dealing with grief and sadness has been helped by giving it a voice and space. I wrote

*poetry and I did artwork and imaging. If I came across something that I found
really difficult, putting it down in painting helped me to understand what
I was feeling.*

Art is a creative expression of sensations at the edge of people's awareness. In
painting or poetry we can express feelings even if we have no language for
it. It is an outlet. A dialogue can start with wondering about the form of art;
its rhythm, shape, and colours. Sometimes, just the thought about what one
would express in artwork can open a bridge when a client is stuck.

*One of us suggested to a client that she might consider expressing her feelings
in painting. When she came back the next week, she didn't want to paint, but
she had thought about what she could paint if she did and talking about it set
the ball rolling.*

With or without artwork, reflecting on oneself, acknowledging changes and
personal vulnerability is an important resource towards a fruitful living in the
future, however long.

Intimacy

Not all patients and families need counselling. Intimate relationships can play
an important role in patients' ability to cope or feel 'healed'. Fiona's loyalty
helped Noel along:

*Noel and Fiona enjoyed hill-walking and crosswords. When Noel had a mas-
sive stroke their life changed forever in a second and the two things that they
did together, recreationally, were completely taken from them. Fiona went from
being a wife to becoming a carer. She cared for him for eighteen years. What
kept her going were some of her beliefs and the way that she could square what
had happened.*

*To start off with, Fiona and Noel had a lot of support from outside, but
over time it disappeared and that contributed to life becoming much more
difficult for them. Noel went through a stage where his speech and his walking
improved, but then it all deteriorated quite markedly and they knew it would
never pick up again. During that 'good phase', you could sense the frustration
of this man—that he couldn't get you always to understand what he was saying, that life was very difficult for him—but most of the time it was remarkable
how he accepted his lot.*

*Healing for Noel was having Fiona with him all the time and the sense of
continuity to know that she would stand by him to the end, no matter what.
He had absolute confidence in that and it was rightly placed. Fiona did come
from a family where doing things for each other and looking out for each*

other was part and parcel of what you did. It was part of what made her who she was.

One of the things that Fiona and Noel used to do together was to go out in the car and drive in the country lanes and go to all the places that they had walked. That wasn't painful. They were able to enjoy the countryside and Noel's face lit up when he was driving along. It was a way of continuing to share a little bit of their life. It maintained a connection with what their relationship had been about.

Fiona's example underlines the burden carers may feel, especially when the duration of illness is prolonged and external support tends to fade away. This couple's whole life was turned upside-down by Noel's stroke. Perhaps Fiona felt lonely at times in what became her life's duty, and perhaps Noel may have felt guilty and embarrassed to put such a strain on his spouse. Yet their mutual trust and loyalty was a haven and, in a creative way, they invented new patterns of sharing their life.

Another patient, Stan, managed to grow in adversity, thanks to intimacy and the support he found in the natural environment and in small things. Suffering from increasingly severe diabetes, he had had to inject himself for decades and had reached a stage where he had no feeling in his legs or feet. He had to imagine what it was like to stand up and walk in order to be able to do so. With a great sense of self-respect, Stan was continuing to work, write, and paint, and it was almost as if with the physical deterioration his sense of personhood had strengthened. Benedict shared:

Stan has been served by the balm of intimacy with a woman who relates to him intellectually, professionally, and loves him physically despite the fact that his body is wasting away. Being in the relationship without having to hide anything and being totally accepted—which is not for a single second in doubt—confirmed him in the very essence of his being.

Another thing that strikes me about Stan is how he can use the natural environment to sustain himself. He can sit and watch a bird, a plant, and to him that is life-giving. Apparently he receives enormous nourishment and succour from the simplest things. It seems as if the illness has taught him to let go and to remain with the essence of being.

Stan's is a very powerful example of a life that looks like a progressive deterioration from the outside but has been the reverse on the inside. It is almost as if the illness left him with no option but to let go, and doing so has enabled him to embrace other aspects of his being and of the world. Benedict reflected:

In the case of Stan the acceptance and letting go has enabled him to enter into the world of the invisible much more fully. He does not see the woman who is so important to him very much, but the bond between them is enormously sustaining to him. He is much nourished also by music and literature. There is a strong—and he would use this word—spiritual dimension to his hold on life and its meaning. He is uncertain about the nature of the life hereafter or even its existence, but he said recently that because so many invisible things sustain him he finds it a perfectly tenable hypothesis that although invisible, there is a life beyond this life.

Stan has managed the difficult transitions that came with his progressive physical deterioration with the support of an intimate relationship in which he could be totally open and free, the strength and succour he found in the natural environment, his creative painting and writing, music and poetry, and more generally in 'invisible' but not 'unnoticeable' resources. His experience is a case in point for non-religious spiritual resources.

Acceptance

We have seen in the discussion about pain and suffering that although not a necessary condition for acceptance, pain control contributes to it in a similar way to how acceptance and willingness contribute to alleviating the pain (see Chapter 14, 'From being the subject of suffering to an observer of pain'). Louis, one of our informants, says:

Feeling bad about feeling bad is a recipe for getting stuck. Feeling okay about feeling bad allows it to move forward into positive emotions. Instead of sadness can come joy; instead of anxiety, calm; instead of shame, a sense of self-worth and acceptance.

For some the verdict 'terminal' seems to operate a shift from fear, anger, pain, and looking backwards to looking ahead and setting an agenda. And yet what they are looking forward to is their dying. Sometimes people have an astonishing breakthrough that leaves them in an ecstatic state for two or three days. Others find wholeness in depletion, admitting that they are who they are and not who they think they are, for in reality none of us is perfect or complete. Sue, a radiographer and counsellor, commented about a couple whose equanimity inspired her:

Keith and May had a strong religious background, but also a huge amount of caring for each other and an acceptance that death was part of life and that actually they were both very sad, but this was okay. There was no angst, and she came and thanked us all. Their journey was just nice, but it was also pain-free.

Benedict recognised in Arthur a journeying 'from resignation to a more positive acceptance'. Once he knew that he was dying Arthur no longer showed signs of depletion or capitulation: a new resolve had come over him. As Balfour Mount put it:

> Once we accept our givens, we are free to assume an attitude to them; to exercise our options; and to take responsibility for ourselves (Mount, 2003 p. 42).

Acceptance comes through 'choosing *not* to' as well as 'choosing to' in recognising and working with the inevitable. Acceptance of a situation, however bad or challenging, is the key to a response to it. It gives opportunity for clear thought, personal assessment, and valid options bravely taken up. As Carl Jung put it, 'Acceptance is the conscious attitude which accompanies integration'. It is the growing wholeness, coherence, and personal integrity that come from an integration and awareness that enable us to choose. It is not a constant state, but rather a moving between accepting what will happen and the anguish of facing death. Rachel, an oncology counsellor, shared this insight:

> *For many clients, there is a moment in the session where they want to be with the sort of dark, worst-case scenario part of themselves; when they want to think 'How will I manage with losing my independence? Losing my ability to care? How am I going to face leaving my family if I die?'. Then they want to click out of that and be with the resourceful side. There seems to be a mix and match between the two worlds.*

The intensity of the experience demands relief and alternation of moods. Louis Heyse-Moore (2009, p. 118) recognises multiple layers in acceptance as he points out that each stage of the story of a major illness will bring its own threats and needs of acceptance. There will be an oscillation of feelings from anger to relief, from sadness to hope, and back again. The series of threats can arise so fast that little time is available to adapt to and accept the new position. As the threats develop, they can bring back unhealed memories of the past and raise further anxieties that may not be immediately relevant to the present situation. Acceptance sounds easy—but it can be a major challenge itself.

Acceptance can and sometimes also needs to be a mutual experience. We have seen with Stan that being fully accepted by someone just as you are, 'warts and all', is very 'healing'. Lester, on the other hand, missed a matching willingness in his partner to accept his dying (see Chapter 9, 'Flexibility in approach and response'). A willingness to wait, to accept where we are at, to savour what we have, and to let go does not come easily. Michael Mayne writes:

> This is the real test: that of patience, humour, trust, and hope. They can only flourish in a climate of acceptance, a recognition of the value to be found in the willingness to wait, wholly dependent on the matching willingness of those who love you to serve you in Blake's 'minute particulars' of love (Mayne, 2006 p. 79).

This may be why, when patients discover acceptance, all the people around them can be transformed by the experience. This happened for Elizabeth (see Chapter 14, 'From being the subject of suffering to an observer of pain') as Martin Laird writes:

> What brought definitive change for the remaining time before her death was the realization that in this very silence there was communion with all people, a loving solidarity with all humanity. The awareness of this was seamlessly united with her awareness of God. This realization expressed itself—even while bedridden—as self-forgetful, loving attentiveness to all whom she met. Health-care professionals, family, and friends arrived to help her and left feeling helped by her…She didn't mean to give, and they didn't intend to receive. But the more she was able to surrender to the loving silence at the centre of her pain, the more she was a vehicle of this loving silence. (Laird, 2006 pp. 108–109)

Practising meditation, Elizabeth noticed an additional 'spiritual' fruit; a sense of connectedness which seemed to include all at her bedside and beyond. Such has been the case for Sophie (see Chapter 7, 'Interdependence and mutual impact'), the young cancer patient who lifted everyone up and indeed for Sara (see Chapter 12, 'Death and dying') who was an inspiration to so many others, even when she became skeletal and blind. For all of them, there was a mutuality between cared-for and carer. The presence of courage, trust, and hope, which are not necessarily related to any particular faith tradition, seems to enhance—or be derived from?—acceptance. As one of our informants said, all resources spill into acceptance!

Acknowledgements

Text extracts from Laird, M., *Into the silent land. The practice of contemplation*, Darton, Longman and Todd, London, UK, Copyright © 2006 Wales Literary Agency, Inc. and Laird, M., *Into the Silent Land: A Guide to the Christian Practice of Contemplation*, Oxford University Press, Inc. New York, USA, Copyright © 2006, by permission of Wales Literary Agency, Inc., Darton, Longman and Todd, and Oxford University Press, USA.

Text extracts from Mayne, M., *The Enduring Melody*, Darton, Longman and Todd, London, UK, Copyright © 2006, reproduced with permission from Darton, Longman and Todd publishers.

References

Bauby, J.-D. 2007. *Le Scaphandre et le Papillon*. Paris: Robert Laffont.

Ferrucci, P. 1982. *What We May Be*. Wellingborough: Turnstone Press.

Glouberman, D. 1989. *Life Choices and Life Changes Through Imagework: the Art of Developing Personal Vision*. London: Unwin Hyman.

Hayes, R. J., Smith, P. G., Carpenter, L., *et al.* 1990. Bristol Cancer Help Centre. Lancet, **336**, 1185–1188.

Heyse-Moore, L. 2009. *Speaking of Dying. a Practical Guide to Using Counselling Skills in Palliative Care*. London and Philadelphia: Jessica Kingsley Publishers.

Johnson, R. A. 1986. *Inner Work*. New York: Harper San Francisco.

Kabat-Zinn, J. 1990. *Full Catastrophe Living: Using the Wisdom of your Body and Mind to Face Stress, Pain and Illness*. New York, Delacorte.

Kabat-Zinn, J. 2003. Mindfulness-based interventions in context: past, present, and future. Clinical Psychology, **10**, 144–156.

Keating, T. 2003. *Invitation to Love—The Way to Christian Contemplation*. New York: Continuum.

Laird, M. 2006. *Into the Silent Land. The Practice of Contemplation*. London: Darton, Longman & Todd.

Mayne, M. 2006. *The Enduring Melody*. London: Darton, Longman & Todd.

Mount, B. M. 2003. Existential suffering and the determinants of healing. European Journal of Palliative Care, **10**, 40–42.

Part 5

The next step

Chapter 15

The next step?

As we near the end of this book, we are reminded of the question asked by our diarist, Veronica, as she approached her death: 'What will be the next step for me?'. Perhaps it is a question we should all ask, especially as it is likely to become so pertinent for us when we experience the passing of our own loved ones and friends and consider our own personal experience of grief.

Looking forward for some will mean facing death, for others a continuing and challenging future. Having confronted many issues, the questions facing patients recorded earlier 'Who am I?' and 'What am I?' may be changed to become 'Who am I now?' and 'What can I be?' and only the future can produce an answer. Veronica recorded in her diary 18 months into her journey with a recurring cancer:

> Where am I on this journey? Who am I now? What do I need to do to travel further, explore deeper?
>
> I feel I have let go of my fears of illness and death, but I cannot quite trust myself in this. What will happen if I really conclude that I have worked through the fear and pain and can let it go? It was there for so long, to teach me, to keep me working things out, being challenged. I don't need it any longer. It has served its purpose well.
>
> What is the next stage about then? 'Growing in wisdom' can only be through experience and consciousness. Going deep into the experience—allowing whatever comes up to be there.

She and many others advise us that the next major challenge awaiting the patient is that of further acceptance of what is and what will be.

Courage is supposed to be grace under pressure,
but it is really composure in the face of inevitability,
being strong not just when the odds favour you,
but when they most decidedly do not.

Philip Gould

Reproduced with permission from Gould, P., *When I Die: Lessons from the Death Zone*, Atom, an imprint of Little, Brown Book Group, London, UK, Copyright © 2012.

The last great adventure

A 92-year old mother, having suffered a stroke, said to her children: 'Death is the last great adventure'. The Latin root of this word, 'adventurus', refers to 'what is about to happen'. It is associated with a sense of the unknown, of risk and uncertainty, and with a rollercoaster of supportive and challenging experiences. Unlike sudden death, or even the gradual effects of dementia, chronic and life-threatening illness allow time to prepare, and the stories in this book suggest that when the journey can be expressed and shared, there may be a sense of adventure in dying; a time of opportunity and challenge. Michael Mayne (2006) affirms the importance of companionship on this journey, but also reminds us of the challenge to the companion in terms of patience and courage. They are not only coping with the patient's feelings of diminishment, but they are also confronted by their own.

We have noted how, as we face the inevitability of death in due course, denial can be a coping strategy for the patient and carers to deal with fears, emotions, and the loss of drive in the face of the unknown. Such pretence can also be the result of a fear of upsetting the other and a desire to protect them. Attitudes of mutual protection can, however, be a disguised protection against our own fear of facing the truth and being upset by the other's reaction. Avoiding these issues can be a cause of awkwardness and discomfort in each other's presence and it is our experience that giving permission and facilitating these difficult conversations can be very enabling. Fear of death or the process towards it is common, but it can be gently dealt with by careful support and encouragement by doctors, psychologists, clergy, carers, and friends. Thus Philip Gould was deeply affected by a statement of consultant psychiatrist David Sturgeon, who encouraged him to understand that, for many people, if not most, death is the most important time of life. (Gould, 2012; p. 111)

In the hospice world, much care is given to how people, patients, family, and friends experience the end of a life. The circumstances will be endlessly variable according to the nature of the illness, of the people involved, and of the relationships between them. The intention of the 'Liverpool Care Pathway for the Dying' (or LCP as it is commonly called) is to provide and monitor personalised care for patient and family that promotes their comfort and well-being at the end of life, physically, emotionally, socially, and spiritually. It is now widely used, not only in hospices but also in hospitals and medical units. When the dying process sets in, the LCP can become a tool to monitor the patient's and the family's comfort and well-being, but far more, it is a way of being that enables life to be lived, even in the very process of dying.

The loss of the future contributes to some patients' overwhelming pain and distress. Facing death, people tend to be reflective about the things that they are losing or will miss out on in the future. They think of things and events that they will not experience such as the spring blossoms in the garden, a child's wedding, the birth of a grandchild. Alice, a hospice chaplain, told us of how she helped people to bridge the gap to an uncertain future by allowing them to mark a significant occasion with a ritual.

> *Doreen's son was divorced and he was getting married again. She'd never liked his first wife and was absolutely delighted he was getting married again. He had three children and his wife-to-be had three children and Doreen was over the moon for them. The wedding was planned for September and this was springtime, so they brought the wedding forward a little bit but, because of her terminal condition, it didn't look as if Doreen was going to make it. She was getting depressed, and I was asked to see what we could do.*
>
> *What we did in the end was to have a ceremony in the chapel in the hospice where I dedicated the rings and where the patient was able to give her formal approval of how happy she was that they were going to get married. They all dressed up in their wedding gear and we had a reception for them in the garden room.*

Doreen wanted to be part of something she really approved of, but because of her terminal condition it was very unlikely that she would be able to. The little ceremony Alice devised allowed Doreen to express her approval of her son's marriage.

Patients cannot easily imagine what life will be like when they are no longer here. As a result Chloe, a therapist, was taken by surprise when Helen, a 40-year-old woman asked: 'When I'm dead will I still be a mother?'.

> *Helen was writing letters to her children—they were aged seven and eleven—and she wanted these letters to be opened by them when they reached the age of eighteen. We had a moving encounter.*
>
> *Helen: I can't read them to my family because they're too close, yet I need to know that these letters are okay. Can I read them to you?*
>
> *[Chloe: I was thinking to myself 'I'm really not sure I have the strength to do this' but I knew I had to say 'yes' of course.]*
>
> *Helen: I can't promise I won't cry while I'm reading them to you.*
>
> *Chloe: I can't promise you I won't cry while I'm listening to them.*
>
> *And that is exactly what happened. At the end Helen said: 'What did you think?' They were just lovely. And as if I would say anything other than they were perfect, because she was their mum, I said: 'You've signed them 'With love from your mother', and that feels terribly formal'.*

> Helen: By the time they reach the age of eighteen, my husband may have remembered and they might call someone else 'Mum'. But I want them to know that I was their mother.

> This is when Helen asked 'Will I still be a mother?', as if she wanted some reinforcement that she would be.

Helen's thoughtfulness to project herself in her children's future and how they would be when they read the letter is touching. Helen wrestled with her sense of her own life coming to an end and how this affected the reciprocity in the relationships with her nearest and dearest. There were things she could not share with her daughters while alive, so she projected herself beyond her death to when her daughters would have become adults without her being around, in order to complete what she considered to be her role as their mother.

Helen seemed almost to mitigate the pain of the loss of her future by projecting herself into her daughters' future and writing them a letter, as if to make herself go on. Caring professionals have been seen to encourage this process, suggesting that patients make a memory box for their child. Chloe warns of underestimating the pain of making such a memory box. Some people simply do not know where to start. Memories are very personal things, and trying to project oneself into the future can come with a surge of unanticipated grief and pain.

We feel that the decision about making a memory box is best guided by the patient's possible loss or gain. If one expects confusion, guilt, or a surge of grief and pain, the memory box may not be a good idea; a letter may help others to fulfil what they consider to be their obligation to children who cannot yet understand. We would encourage patients to communicate as openly as possible about their intention. If, for instance, the memory box or letter became an escape from personally addressing an issue with a loved one, the survivor might be left to deal with regret and guilt that might have been avoided by talking through the issue together.

If the need for something to remember the patient by lies with the survivors, it might be better that they take the initiative for it themselves. Thus Chloe would have a child make a treasure box about its dying parent, as she did with Cal.

> The box had pictures on it and there were lots of things in there that were around Cal's relationship with his mum. There were things that he felt ought to go in there, that people had said, 'Oh you can put that in your treasure box; that will remind you of Mummy' and things around the funeral. But the things that Cal had put in himself were lovely: a pair of fluffy socks, because Mummy's feet got so cold and she was always wearing fluffy socks; a pair of sunglasses

because there was a funny story attached to Mummy losing sunglasses and where they'd been found. Then there was a tiny little sealable plastic bag with a piece of tissue in with the last few drops of mummy's perfume.

Cal had chosen these things and I asked, 'Do you smell it often?'. As a nine-year old he said, 'I don't open it, because I know the smell will go. So I need to save it for special occasions'. We talked about what would constitute a special occasion, which would be when he was really sad and he wanted to remember Mum.

Treasure boxes, letters, and memory boxes can be supportive in maintaining connections, both in life and in death. Still, as with so many of the factors we have discussed, for success of the intervention it is a matter of timing, of tuning and offering the apt suggestion when something prompts us to do so. This makes the point again that people just are so different that anything approaching a 'rule' for what would be good to do is untenable. That may be even more so when we are thinking of what would be helpful to a child. There is something important here about taking really seriously the person-centred idea that only the client or patient can know.

Grief and bereavement

However good the care and the experience of the death, we must recognise that relatives and friends who love the dying person will experience tension, shock, and grief, and subsequently a sense of emptiness and loss. Hospices seek to meet these needs even beyond the death of the patient with ongoing bereavement care. For those left behind, the adjustment to the new circumstances may take months and even years to achieve. For some, the sense of loss can be permanent and tragic, but most people will experience gradual recovery from grief, even if some emotional scars remain. They will be changed and a new life opens up for them. Their hurdle initially lies behind the questions 'What life?' and 'How will I cope?' A painful chapter may have closed, but they may be asking whether the succeeding ones will be any better.

The circumstances of a death can be hugely variable from a gentle departure during sleep to a traumatic accident or violent assault. The nature of the death will affect the bereavement process and the effect it has on those who loved and cared for the deceased. But at its heart and over time, the sense of loss will be generally similar, even if the way it is expressed will vary according to the characteristics of the mourner. However, there are notable situations that could colour the 'normal' process. For instance, the loss of a child can raise deep questions of fairness and appropriateness; the death of a young person in the armed services will present a clash of grief with pride that someone has died on behalf of others, even his country; with suicide, a grief may be tinged or dominated by anger, guilt, or overwhelming shock.

What is very significant for our purposes at this juncture are the attitudes expressed by family, friends, and neighbours towards those grieving the passing of a loved one. Often, after leaving them alone immediately prior to the funeral, there is a flurry of attention in the following weeks, which comes to an end after perhaps a month or two. Those grieving are once again left to themselves. People turn back to their own preoccupations and priorities, which often do not include those who mourn. They in turn are left feeling deserted, lonely, and isolated. This experience tends to come just at the point when they are recovering from the shock of the death and when loving support is most needed. The sense of loss is therefore compounded. Many experience this withdrawal as a sign of the general expectation that they should 'get over' the death and its consequences as if it had never happened. We consider this as an example of communal denial of the far-reaching impact of dying and death.

Whatever the circumstances, the deceased's life has ended and the life of the bereaved continues, but some of the powerful bonds that held them together may be continued, yet in an incomplete way. The grieving person may feel half a person, as if part of them has died too. So while one life is over, what is felt by others can be like a major wound to the heart and spirit. It is hardly surprising therefore that so many bereaved people endure a period of feeling depressed, or what looks like it. They are lost, confused, and confronted without their 'other half' or perhaps their child. Another factor behind this personal wound is that if one lives close to another, relies on another, is committed to another, a mutual dependency develops, with both giving and receiving support, encouragement, and shared practical experience. As such mutual dependency develops over the years, its breaking can be felt as an amputation, as one person known to us described it. Part of her had almost physically been removed. Such a psychological experience is strengthened by the loss of physical contact and intimacy with the beloved, especially in a marriage or partnership. The world seems cold. There is nobody to share oneself with, one's ideas, one's hopes and fears, at the level which these things may require. Touch, warmth, total togetherness bonded by physical and visible love, are lost. Most fear, at least early on, that such closeness has been lost forever. The bereaved feels deeply bereft. The informant quoted earlier also described it as '…being cut in half. Not only has my husband died, I feel I have too. Will I ever live again?'. Such deep feelings of desolation in some people begin to soften during the first year; but for many the timescale is much longer and can be, like for Queen Victoria, lifelong. Their personal resources are damaged; they cannot move on.

It is in this dark period that some begin to recognise a powerful sense of closeness to the person who died. They talk to them; they go to the grave to meet them; they sit in their chair, or even cook their favourite meal and lay a place at the table for them. Some of the most eccentric expressions of pining can indicate a lack of acceptance of the new circumstances, but they can also indicate a sense of continuance and may not be a denial of the death or a trick of the mind, but just a longing for the presence of someone lost. It could be an awareness that the deceased is there in spirit. The phenomenon of searching is far from uncommon, especially in the early days of bereavement. In our experience, in most cases this should not be denied or minimised by those who seek to help the grieving, but, if it is comforting to them, accepted as a sign of adjustment to new circumstances.

Many people need help to cope with this powerful form of loneliness and this is where generous and understanding members of the family and circle of friends can help. But they must be careful not to pressurise the person or to try to move them on faster than they can manage. It is vital for their future well-being that changes occur in the grieving process at the pace of the person mourning, which may not be that of the helpers. It is a particular support if the helpers knew the deceased, as this will help them more closely to identify with what the loved one is going through. The deceased can be talked about and appreciated first hand.

In time, many bereaved will begin to live again. They may start to go out in the evenings, rejoin clubs and groups, and even stay away at friends and go on holiday. Some begin new friendships that meet some of the needs associated with deep loneliness. Such relationships can become close and become a subject of great happiness, not only for those concerned but also their families. When a new-found partnership begins, this should not necessarily be seen as a denial of what had been; it can be an affirmation of what was and is. It is a new experience desired and valued, and although it will almost certainly be different, it will nevertheless be fulfilling and restorative. A new zest for life can be discovered.

While most people in bereavement are supported by family and friends—some sadly are not—some may need the gift of bereavement support by volunteers or professionals. Bereavement counsellors have the skills to help the client develop a balanced memory and response to what has happened to them. The deep feelings of the bereaved person, frequently unrecognised or even resented, can be accepted and worked on so that their sting can be drawn.

While the previous marriage or partnership may have had its difficulties and sometimes major ones, when it is broken it is still felt as a grievous loss and is identified outwardly as such. However, subconscious resentment and anger may exist and continue undermining the authentic memory of the relationship. In such circumstances, grief is likely to be extended. Professional counsellors can assist in the discovery and acceptance of realities, and this can have the effect of bringing a new sense of peace and hope.

It is obvious that grief is a painful experience but it need not necessarily be destructive. It may well require empathy and understanding from those around the mourner. With support and time, a new life can develop and the experiences of the past can make their own contribution to it. A painful chapter may have closed, but the story of a life continues.

In conclusion

The writing of this book coincided with the final journey of two dear relatives, one for each of us. It has been humbling to walk alongside them, blindfolded, while trying to write about how to help people live their dying. It served to prove—if we needed any convincing—that people die alone and in a very personal way, just as they live, and that the best we can do is to be there at the door if and when they can, or choose to, open it. This personal experience for both of us has put our writing into perspective: the process of dying is and remains a huge and inevitable mystery. People do die alone and unaccompanied, but we may be with them to the very threshold.

We have extensively commented on the powerful and unexpected changes that life-altering and life-threatening illness may not only bring to patients but also their families and those who love and serve their needs as carers. The list of potential losses is long, including family style and equilibrium, friends, participation in outside activities, hobbies, and holidays among many others. The situation for all concerned is tough; but we also see how it can bring the best out of people, opening them to new opportunities and risks. The experience tests us all—our strength, our character, and spirituality—and from it there is real potentiality for growth along the path on which lies death. After all, it may therefore be confirmed in everyday experience that in life is death, and through dying, we find life, love, and true personhood. For what more could we ask?

We end this book with Veronica, our diary writer, who wrote down her dream. This telling story gives a voice to her journey…and ours.

I had this dream…

I am a sea otter. I swim, explore, dive, fish, collect sea urchins which are delicious food. Life in the sea is free, wide and open, exciting and frightening. When we were young and fit we swam and played—we thought we would play forever. We were invincible—our thick coats shone, our eyes were bright and innocent, we swam freely and joyfully.

When we got a bit older, some of us got sick. Others were frightened. We no longer felt immortal. The future was no longer certain. It did not stretch out into the distance as far as the eye could see.

But not everyone was frightened. There were some wise old—and not-so-old—otters about, and their words enveloped me, held me, freed me. Let go, they said—certainty is just an illusion. Everything is impermanence. Leave behind your attachments to security and certainty. We cannot know the future. It does not exist. What does exist is each moment—when we feel joy, anger, pain, bliss in this moment. That is real. How can we be sure the next moment will happen? If we cannot be sure, then the wise otter knows that letting go into that bliss, that pain, that moment is all we can do.

Otters live in families. We swim together, fish together, play together. We have friends and families and lovers. We are taught that there are rules and our futures will be in danger if we break the rules. Otters will be angry in the future; otters will be hurt; otters will reject us in the future. We will be hurt.

But what if there is no future, and we followed the rules, thinking there was? Each precious moment of bliss or pain, of deep exciting uncertainty would be lost, and could not be regained.

So the wise otter learns to trust the moment, love the moment—the future will be one, or ten or a million moments lived in bliss and pain.

References

Gould, P. 2012. *When I Die. Lessons from the Death Zone.* London: Atom, an imprint of Little, Brown.

Mayne, M. 2006. *The Enduring Melody.* London, Darton, Longman & Todd.

Postscript

When Catherine Proot and Michael Yorke kindly invited me to contribute a postscript to their book my first thought was 'Why me?' Though flattered to be asked, I do not have a counselling or clinical background and therefore felt that I could not possibly do justice to this book. But after explanation from Catherine that they were hoping that I would be able to affirm that their book was very much in line with Dame Cicely Saunders' thinking and philosophy, I agreed to write this postscript. So I picked up the book and began to read...

As I delved deeper into the book it became clear to me that several of Dame Cicely's messages to us in the early days of the hospice movement were echoing across the pages.

The plea for 'openness to patients, families, those who come to learn and ourselves'—the inspiration for the founding of St Christopher's Hospice in 1967—is very evident from the start of the book. For the book is clear, both in content and in layout, making it easy to read and accessible to anyone who might be affected by a terminal illness: patients, carers including both family and friends, and professionals too. And what makes the book so 'open', so accessible, is the use of stories. Concepts are introduced and explained clearly but then the 'proof of the pudding'—a personal reflection or story from family member, patient, or a member of the professional team—lifts the book to another level. I remember clearly how Dame Cicely would always illustrate her lectures with simple but beautiful slides and her words: 'Let the patient tell the story'.

As I read on, I was reminded of her support and, indeed, insistence when we first produced our magazine, *The Hospice Bulletin*, that we should publish the stories of hospice and palliative care teams and individuals that were just starting out—to give them a voice; their work was not important enough at that time to attract the academic journals. No one can presume Dame Cicely's reaction to this book but it is my guess that she might well have enjoyed hearing the patient's voice, which comes through so clearly.

Moreover, always a stickler for clear and accurate text, I think that she might have appreciated the practical aspects of this book. I still have some cards written by her—she would write to every member of staff on the anniversary of their joining the hospice—describing what she liked about the information service that we delivered; words such as:

- reaching out
- openness
- networking
- collecting people's experiences
- accurate and up-to-date information
- friendliness and approachability.

To me, each of these words and phrases could equally describe this remarkable book. It reaches out to the lay public and to professionals, it is open and accessible, written in an engaging and reader-friendly way, there are clear explanations, copious references and it is definitely a repository of people's experiences.

At a personal level, having watched too many close friends and family approaching their own deaths in past two years, I have found the book enormously helpful. The resilience and courage of the people whose stories are told is impressive. We all have something to learn.

Avril Jackson
for 31 years head of the Hospice Information
Service at St Christopher's
September 2013

Index